ACUPUNCTURE

IN THE SAME SERIES:

Principles of Aromatherapy
Cathy Hopkins

Principles of Buddhism
Kulananda

Principles of Chinese Medicine
Angela Hicks

Principles of Chinese Herbal Medicine
John Hicks

Principles of Colonic Irrigation
Jillie Collings

Principles of the Enneagram
Karen Webb

Principles of Fasting
Leon Chaitow

Principles of Feng Shui
Simon Brown

Principles of Hypnotherapy
Vera Peiffer

Principles of Native American Spirituality
Dennis Renault and Timothy Freke

Principles of NLP
Joseph O'Connor and Ian McDermott

Principles of Nutritional Therapy
Lina Lazarides

Principles of Paganism
Vivianne Crowley

Principles of your Psychic Potential
David Lawson

Principles of Psychotherapy
Brice Avery

Principles of Reflexology
Nicola Hall

Principles of Self-Healing
David Lawson

Principles of Shiatsu
Chris Jarmey

Principles of Stress Management
Vera Peiffer

Principles of Tarot
Evelyne and Terry Donaldson

Principles of Yoga
Sara Martin

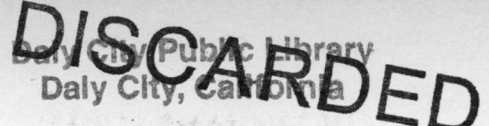

THORSONS
PRINCIPLES
OF

ACUPUNCTURE

ANGELA HICKS

Thorsons
An Imprint of HarperCollins*Publishers*

W

Thorsons
An Imprint of HarperCollins*Publishers*
77 – 85 Fulham Palace Road,
Hammersmith, London W6 8JB
1160 Battery Street
San Francisco, California 94111–1213

Published by Thorsons 1997

3 5 7 9 10 8 6 4

A catalogue record for this book
is available from the British Library

ISBN 0 7225 3409 4

Printed and bound in Great Britain by
Caledonian International Book Manufacturing, Glasgow

CONTENTS

Author's Note   vii
Introduction   ix

1 Who Has Acupuncture Treatment?   1
2 Why Do We Become Ill?   14
3 What Theory is Used to Make a Diagnosis?   30
4 How is a Diagnosis Carried Out?   55
5 When I Have Treatment What Will it be Like?   72
6 How are Children Treated With Acupuncture?   92
7 What Other Forms of Acupuncture Treatment
  are Available?   97
8 What Guidelines Can I Follow to Help me
  Stay Healthy?   108
9 Where Can I Go For Treatment?   114

Useful Addresses   119
Index   121

AUTHOR'S NOTE

This book is written as an informative guide to acupuncture and is not meant as a self-help book for treatment.

As with my previous book, *Principles of Chinese Medicine*, I have written this book in the feminine pronoun throughout. This is not meant as any slight to the 50 per cent of the population that are male. It is merely that I have had to make a choice and the English language does not yet provide a neutral pronoun that I could use. I have also capitalized all Chinese medicine terminology in order to differentiate them from standard English terms.

My thanks to all of the people who by their contributions have helped me to write this book.

First, thank you to all of my patients who talked with me about their experiences of acupuncture. Thanks also to the patients of Sally Blades, Judith Clark, Di Cook, Claire Cromarty, Jill Glover, Celene Kershen, Stella King, Salvador March, Carey Morgan, Gail Newton, Alison West, Penny Wilson and Billie Wray. The names of all patients have been changed to protect confidentiality. Of these practitioners, Alison, Billie, Judith, Sally, Stella and Di also answered my probing questions in relation to carrying out diagnoses and treatments.

Secondly, thanks to those practitioners who helped me with essential information that I've used in this book, especially Beth Soderstrom who talked to me about the treatment of drug abusers, Celene Kershen who discussed the treatment of children, Geraldine Worthington who treats animals and David Mayor who uses electro-acupuncture.

Thanks also to all those who have helped me by reading through this book, most notably Judith Clark, as well as Sophie Hayes and Peter Mole.

Finally, my thanks and love to John, my husband, who is always so supportive and loving.

INTRODUCTION

O ne of the most common questions that I am asked about acupuncture is, 'Does it work?' Before we address this important question we also need to ask, 'What is acupuncture?'

Acupuncture has been a complete system of treatment for at least 2,000 years. At this time a book called *The Yellow Emperor's Classic of Internal Medicine* was written. This book is still used by practitioners today. Over the past 2,000 years acupuncture has continued to evolve and develop – that it has survived for so long is a convincing tribute to its effectiveness.

Acupuncture treatment is carried out by inserting a few fine needles into points on the body. The effect of the needles is to restore the balance of the patients' energy and thereby improve their health. Acupuncture treatment both addresses specific symptoms and has an overall effect whereby patients often 'feel better in themselves'.

Our original question was, 'Does it work?' Many of the people who have already had treatment have experienced that it is a beneficial treatment. Research confirms this to be true.

In the winter of 1995, one of the largest surveys of acupuncture patients to date was carried out in the United States. Five

x hundred and seventy five acupuncture patients from six clinics answered a 29-question survey into the effects of acupuncture.

The result was that an amazing 90 per cent of patients reported the disappearance or improvement of their symptoms after treatment! In addition, 91 per cent said that they were extremely satisfied or very satisfied with their acupuncturist. Eighty-eight per cent liked the treatment and 70 per cent thought the cost was extremely satisfactory or very satisfactory even though they weren't reimbursed by their medical insurance.

Most of the patients were between 30 and 60 years old and 75 per cent were women. Of the patients who filled in the questionnaire 79 per cent said they now use fewer medical drugs, 71 per cent said they had avoided surgery and 84 per cent said they needed to see their doctor less frequently.

You may not know that acupuncture is one of the fastest growing treatments in the Western world. This survey tells us why – it achieves remarkable results! For further evidence of its effectiveness we can look at some of the striking findings of other research which has been carried out in China and the West.

One study was carried out on 2,041 pregnant women in China. These women were between 29 and 40 weeks pregnant and all had a mal-positioned or 'breech' baby. Treatment consisted of heating an acupuncture point at the end of the little toe. Of those treated 90 per cent were corrected.

Of the 90 per cent, 86 per cent were corrected after only 1–4 treatments and the remaining 14 per cent after 5–10 treatments. Often the mother could feel the baby moving when treatment was applied. This 90 per cent response compares with a 60 per cent spontaneous change under normal circumstances.

Another research project, this time in England, was carried out at the Churchill Hospital in Oxford in 1986 and was subsequently written up in the medical journal the *Lancet*. In this study, acupuncture was carried out on patients who had had disabling breathlessness for at least five years. A placebo group was also given treatment on non-acupuncture points.

After only three weeks the acupuncture group showed significant improvement – they both felt better and could walk for six minutes over longer distances than the placebo group. There was a conspicuous 49 per cent improvement in the real acupuncture group as opposed to a 19 per cent improvement in the placebo group. Two of the placebo group became envious of patients in the real acupuncture group as it was clear that they were making such good progress!

Acupuncture has been widely used in the treatment of pain. A study was carried out in 1987 on 43 women with painful periods. One group had real acupuncture, a second group had placebo acupuncture, a third group had no treatment and a fourth group had visits with a physician but no treatment.

The acupuncture group showed a 90.9 per cent improvement, the placebo acupuncture group 36.4 per cent, the no treatment group 18.2 per cent and the fourth group 10 per cent. There was a 41 per cent reduction of painkillers in the acupuncture group with no change in painkillers for the other groups.

Although these studies all speak for themselves, the people best equipped to talk to us about acupuncture are the patients themselves. We will meet seven of them – Edna, Paul, Marion, Janie, Anita, Karen and Rose – in the next chapter.

This book will also answer many important questions about acupuncture and provide us with an overview of its main theory. As well as how a diagnosis is carried out, it will also cover what it is like to be treated and what causes us to become ill in the first place. We will discuss the treatment of children and some unusual forms of treatment such as the treatment of animals, electro-acupuncture, ear acupuncture and a new treatment which can help drug abusers.

PRINCIPLES OF ACUPUNCTURE

WHO HAS ACUPUNCTURE TREATMENT?

When I decided to write this book I asked acupuncture friends and colleagues if they knew of any patients who would be willing to talk to me about their experiences of having treatment. The result was an overwhelming number of patients keen to tell me how acupuncture had helped them. Some talked to me because they enjoyed telling their stories. Others wanted to recommend it to other people who have health problems. Most were keen to speak because they thought acupuncture deserved more publicity.

In this chapter I will introduce you to a cross section of these people and tell you what they said about their experiences of acupuncture. As the book progresses we will also hear from some of the other patients I have talked to while writing this book.

WHO HAS ACUPUNCTURE?

The patients I talked to had gone for acupuncture treatment with a vast range of problems. I divided them into six broad categories.

The first category was made up of people who had gone for treatment with *some form of ache or pain*. They included people with joint conditions – from rheumatoid arthritis or osteoarthritis to shoulder problems, pain following accidents or trauma and also pain from headaches and migraines.

The second group was a very different kind of pain – emotional pain. These I would call *'mental-spiritual' conditions.* Often patients had more difficulty verbalizing these problems. 'I didn't want to go on any more,' one patient told me. 'I had a loss of confidence and was near a breakdown,' said another. One patient described being depressed, whilst several had severe anxiety. One other described the support acupuncture had given her during a difficult phase in her life, and another described the 'fine tuning' it gave him for his emotional problems. Many patients who came for more physical conditions described the additional changes that acupuncture brought to their mental or emotional state and hence their life in general.

A third group of patients were those with *physical problems.* These included people with digestive conditions – bloating up after eating, loose bowels or constipation, hiatus hernia and vomiting to name a few. Other illnesses treated were gynaecological problems, lung ailments, urinary problems, heart conditions and thyroid disorders.

A fourth category were those who had *acute infections* such as coughs and colds treated whilst undergoing acupuncture treatment for other conditions. Also included in this group are those who had other 'viral' conditions such as post-viral syndrome which is so common these days, and glandular fever.

The fifth category was made up of patients who had *severe long-term chronic illnesses.* Some patients went for treatment with problems which benefited greatly from acupuncture while they continued to have strong support from Western medicine – one patient had had breast lumps removed and used acupuncture to help her through the trauma, another patient was helped through attacks of Lupus, which had previously caused stiffness and pain all over her body, and an insulin-dependent diabetic found acupuncture helped him to maintain his health. Other illnesses were chronic skin complaints, long-standing exhaustion and one patient with 'Ramsey Hart' Syndrome which is a rare condition of severe degenerative paralysis.

Finally, the sixth group was made up of patients who had acupuncture to *remain healthy*. A few came to treatment because they were merely curious, some came because they wished to positively enhance their health. Many other patients had originally come to treatment with an illness. This had now been cured but they continued to be treated every 1–3 months in order to stay well.

THE SPECTRUM OF PATIENTS

In this chapter I have picked out patients with many different complaints. Edna had a shoulder problem, Paul went for treatment with migraines, Marion had a complete loss of confidence when her job changed and Janie had many severe problems which included polycystic ovarian syndrome, severe night sweats, exhaustion and high blood pressure. Anita, a 19-year-old, had treatment for glandular fever whilst Karen went after having breast lumps removed and had the support of acupuncture treatment during chemotherapy. Finally, Rose went because she wanted an 'MOT' and to keep well.

EDNA'S STORY

'I'm usually tough,' Edna told me, 'I worked in the mills for 40 years or so and you learn that if a problem comes along you either do something about it or forget it.'

Edna is 76 years old and has lived in Lancashire all of her life. 'I went for treatment because I'd had a frozen shoulder for six

4 months. It appeared within a day and a half and I still don't know where it came from. I was restricted in every way and I couldn't bear to spend the rest of my life in pain. I couldn't comb my hair, pull out a drawer or grip anything – the pain just shot from my shoulder to my thumb. I was so desperate that life wasn't worth living. I'd got very down and depressed, it was shocking.

'I went in January and even after the first treatment it eased. After three times the difference was amazing and it got better and better! Now I can use it for anything and I've even painted and decorated the kitchen. I do get a very slight ache still if I use an area behind my shoulder but I don't normally feel it. I've really gone back to being how I was. I'd also had a bad back from a fall and that got better too – I've never had the pain since. Now I say, don't be put off by acupuncture, you don't know until you've tried it. Whatever it cost me it's worth every penny.'

PAUL'S STORY

Paul also had pain before having acupuncture treatment but his came from migraines. Paul is 56 years old and comes from outside Cardiff. He manages a laundry. Here he tells his story.

'I didn't go for treatment with any belief in a cure. I decided to try acupuncture as there weren't any other treatments left! I'd tried homoeopathy, reflexology, aromatherapy and osteopathy before I went for acupuncture. I'd also taken many painkillers. I no longer need to take painkillers.

'I was having migraines. I'd get pains in the right-hand side of my head, over the right eye, and they'd last anything from two or three days to a week. They varied in severity and were either "uncomfortable" or "very uncomfortable" or "evil". The evil ones appeared once every three months. Now the migraines have effectively gone.

'I was going for treatment once a fortnight for two months and there was such a vast improvement in the headaches that after four or five visits I thought, "I'm OK now". My practitioner had warned me I wasn't completely better. After one month I started getting the migraines back. I put up with it for a while then I had one that lasted for five weeks. It was terrible. I finally went back for more treatment and my headache went the next day. I've been having treatment now for six months and still go regularly. I occasionally have a migraine but only about once every three months.

'My circumstances are no different and my job is still as pressurized as before but now I'm much more relaxed – other people have commented on it as well. I believe tension brought it on. People tell me I'm much less "sparky", aggressive and demanding – I think I'm the same.

'I was neutral as to whether I believed or disbelieved in treatment but I really don't believe that the fact that I got better was psychosomatic. I now wonder what else acupuncture can do and what the possibilities are.'

Paul knew that his migraines were caused by tension at work. The pace and pressure of life nowadays causes many people to have similar problems.

MARION'S STORY

Marion is a nurse. She is 48 years old and has two grown-up children. She lives in Surrey. She is also the proud grandmother of a three-and-a-half-year old.

'It all started when I was sent on a course in children's nursing. Before that I'd been working in the Accident and Emergency Centre of a hospital and enjoyed it. I'd got worried when I was training to be a nurse but never this bad. I thought I would have a nervous breakdown and I was frightened because no one could understand me or explain my symptoms and nothing anyone said could make me feel better.

'Really I was afraid of the essays I had to do. I had sleepless nights and would be thinking about college work. I'd wake early in a hot sweat so I'd get up early but then I couldn't concentrate when I got up. I was desperate to get my work done but I couldn't. If I was at work I was more at ease as I wasn't thinking about my essays. I got loose bowels in the mornings, I was smoking excessively and my food wouldn't go down. I couldn't talk about anything except my fear of essays. I went to the doctor. He wanted to give me a drug called Propranolol. I knew it wouldn't cure me so I said I didn't want it.

'One day I talked to a colleague and told her I'd lost all of my confidence and she said, "Why not try acupuncture?"

'I couldn't believe it when my acupuncturist understood what was going on. Then when I had treatment I could feel the needles working straight away. I could feel movement in my temples and the side of my neck. I didn't even think about them as needles. I was surprised they were so small and I felt nothing sharp going in me. I really enjoy having treatment. I think of it as my time when I know I'm going to have a relaxing hour. After the first few treatments I felt as if I was wrapped in cotton wool. I went in frightened and came out with a smile on my face.

'On the whole now I'm back to normal. I'm still doing the course but I'm not aware of the amount of work involved and I've only got three more essays to do. My outlook about going back to Accident and Emergency is now different – I used to be frightened that I couldn't cope, now I know I could. I'm eating and sleeping and my bowels are fine, I'm even not smoking as much. I'd never have believed it. In fact since having acupuncture I'm able to relax more in my own time. Sometimes I even sing when I'm coming home in the car.'

Marion was first treated at an acupuncture college by a third-year student who was supervised by a faculty member.

Janie is an acupuncture student who is now treating her own patients under supervision. Over her years at the college Janie has gone through a complete metamorphosis. She now tells us what happened to her. She is 31 years old and lives in Staines in Middlesex.

'I was already an acupuncture student when I went for treatment with my practitioner. I was so unwell in myself that finally I decided that I'd better put my money where my mouth was and have some. Now I can truly say that acupuncture has changed my life and it's also given me life. Before I had treatment I didn't realize how ill I was and therefore what limitations I had.

'I had "polycystic ovarian syndrome" which means that my ovaries were covered in cysts. I also had terrible night sweats, heavy periods and period pain, exhaustion, obesity, migraines, many food allergies, chronic sinusitis and my blood pressure was high. I found it difficult to get up before 11 o'clock in the morning; it was like swimming to the surface of a sea of treacle. The list of my symptoms was endless.

'I had become very ill when I was 17. I had terrible period pains and clots and very heavy, irregular periods. I never had a normal period. Now they're lovely! At that time I had an operation where they stripped the ovaries and removed the cysts. The operation didn't help as I was put on medication that caused me just as many symptoms. Later the lining of my womb built up so much I felt as if I was passing a six month foetus through a non-dilated cervix. I went to the top people and they couldn't help me.

'My experience shows how far down you can go and still come up again. I no longer have any of my symptoms. The acupuncture is amazing! People now don't recognize me, I'm a different person. I've lost weight and I try to explain that it's a

8   reflection of my well-being. It's like being reborn and I probably get boring talking about it. It's the most incredible thing that's happened to me.

'I had a scan in the summer holidays and my ovaries were normal. The chap who did the scan was amazed. I want to go to the specialists and say, 'See'. They told me I was infertile and now I'm sure I'm not. I haven't taken any pills for eighteen months. Before I was on hormones and painkillers and took low-dose antibiotics for acne for eight years. I'm now always in bed before midnight – it used to be around 3 o'clock in the morning. I also eat properly which I didn't do before.

'I feel different emotionally and spiritually in every way. It's like having had a wet suit on and being liberated. I feel a lightness and freedom and a release. Sometimes I don't think people are aware of the scope of acupuncture. I feel as if everything is possible in my life now!'

ANITA'S STORY

Anita is 19 years old. She lives in Bolton and works as a customer service representative in a video store.

'I was never a sick child and was really healthy until I got glandular fever. I know the person I caught it from. I borrowed a pen and chewed it. I think I was run down at the time from a lot of schoolwork. The onset was very sudden. It came on in November when I was 14 years old.

'When I had the glandular fever my bones felt tender and sore and my muscles were stiff and tight. I had a very sore throat and swollen glands. When I went to the acupuncturist I was very depressed with it and I was also extremely lethargic, anxious and forgetful. I'd lost a lot of weight as I didn't have the energy to eat. People had thought I was playing up as I didn't want to go to school. In all, the glandular fever went on for about three years. It finished just before my A levels.

'Mum made me the appointment with the acupuncturist. She had gone to get help for a frozen shoulder so she picked up the phone and made me an appointment too.

'The first time I went for acupuncture treatment it had a very calming effect and I felt the energy going all around my body. The high lasted a couple of days and the panic attacks and anxiety went and the depression lifted as well. I went every week for three weeks then every two weeks for three months. In the end my practitioner was treating me for my overall health. About two months after treatment began I could deal with things better and I found I had mental and physical energy. I'd been thirsty and that eased almost straight away and never came back.

'Now I would say that I'm not as selfish and as angry as I used to be. I'm not the centre of the universe any more. I can't explain it. The illness and the treatment have changed me. Being ill for so long gave me lots of time to think about things. To me acupuncture was the best treatment I could have had, it's uplifting and clearing and it's completely natural.'

KAREN'S STORY

Some people come for treatment with a serious illness and acupuncture and Western medicine can mutually support each other. Karen was one such person. She is 42 years old and comes from the north of England. She works as a probation officer.

'I had a really, really stressful year the year before I got breast cancer. Later I read a book about the type of person who gets cancer and I recognized myself. I'd had breast cancer and had the lump removed but the doctors hadn't got it all. It spread to the lymph nodes and was an aggressive type.

'I went on holiday for five weeks to see my sister in Australia. She helped me to sort my head out and made an

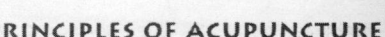

appointment with an acupuncturist there. The acupuncturist gave me the confidence to change and to live. I saw her twice then came back to England. I decided to have chemotherapy and radiation therapy and also decided to get the support of acupuncture again.

'The acupuncture gave me the energy to cope with the chemotherapy and to feel positive about myself. I worked right through the chemotherapy then took a month off work. When I went in for treatment and was really down, acupuncture gave me a lift. I've gone to treatment and wept buckets and come out feeling brighter and more positive about life. Treatment helped me to feel life was worth living.

'Having acupuncture was a massive contrast to the health service. I always felt really positive after acupuncture treatment whereas treatment at the hospital made me feel negative.

'People are really reluctant to believe me when I tell them about acupuncture. They think it's all in my mind. It's magical stuff and you can sort out any problem with it, not just physical ones.'

ROSE'S STORY

Rose lives in Reading and is a retired junior school headmistress. She had acupuncture in order to stay healthy – a good reason for having treatment but one many people don't think about. This is what she has to say about treatment.

'When I first came it was really for an 'MOT' and to find out about acupuncture rather than for any specific problem. I'd heard that acupuncture was a good thing and I liked what I'd heard about it. I did have some little things that I'd never have gone to the doctor with. It was energy more than anything and the time to talk about myself in various ways.

'After the first treatments I didn't really feel any change, then it was the fourth treatment that I really felt cracked it. I'd had a horrendous day and popped down for a treatment. I immediately felt more relaxed. Later on I went to my in-laws who were ill and got home at 11.30pm and still felt wonderful! I went to bed and felt ready to run school for another day. It was like an unblocking of my energy.

'I think the treatment lifted me on to a different level. After treatment I could stay up until 11pm, before I had to go to bed at 8.30pm. I used to sleep heavily on Saturdays and Sundays – a deep, deep sleep, I still retreat sometimes but just to relax – I very rarely sleep.

'I just wish there was a way to get more people to be willing to try it, particularly for tiredness and lack of energy, I think it's a tragedy when people say, "I could never go" or "I'm not brave enough". The image they get is of big needles, not of little fine ones. It really is a problem I think.'

Edna, Marion, Janie, Paul, Anita, Karen and Rose have all benefited from treatment. Although not every patient has as miraculous a result as they did, most people do gain some relief from treatment and acupuncture can deal with a wide range of problems.

SOME OF THE ILLNESSES ACUPUNCTURE CAN HELP

Breathing and lung problems such as asthma; chronic breathlessness; bronchitis; coughs; colds; influenza; hay fever.

Circulatory problems such as angina; chronic heart conditions; high or low blood pressure; palpitations; poor circulation; stroke; thrombosis; varicose veins.

Digestive and bowel complaints such as inflamed gall bladder; gall stones; gastritis; indigestion; nausea; stomach ulcers; vomiting; colitis; constipation; diarrhoea; dysentery; irritable bowel syndrome.

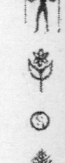

12 **Ear, eye, nose, mouth and throat disorders** such as blurred vision; chronic catarrh; conjunctivitis; deafness; dry eyes; gum problems; nosebleeds; otitis media; sinusitis; sore throats; tinnitus; tonsillitis; toothache.

Emotional and mental conditions such as anxiety; depression; eating disorders; insomnia; panic attacks.

Gynaecological disorders such as heavy periods; hot flushes and other menopausal problems; irregular periods; morning sickness; period pain; premenstrual tension; scanty or no periods; post-natal depression; vaginal discharge.

Joint problems and pain such as back problems; joint injuries or inflammation; headaches; osteoarthritis, rheumatoid arthritis, rheumatism; sciatica; Stills disease.

Neurological problems such as Bell's palsy; epilepsy; multiple sclerosis; neuralgia.

Sudden acute disorders such as the common cold; food poisoning; stomach upsets; influenza; mumps.

Skin conditions such as acne; eczema; psoriasis; urticaria.

Urinary and reproductive problems such as bed wetting; cystitis; impotence; urine retention; incontinence; infertility; kidney stones; prostate conditions.

This list does not cover every single illness that acupuncture can deal with but may expand your view of what it can help. Some people think that acupuncture can only treat certain kinds of complaints. I have heard people say, 'Acupuncture can only treat painful conditions' or at the other extreme, 'It only deals with psychological problems'. In fact it can assist people to become healthier at every level – physically, mentally and spiritually.

A practitioner understands that our body, mind and spirit are inseparable. When Edna had a painful shoulder she became very depressed. When Marion was nervous of writing essays her emotional state affected her digestion and her sleeping.

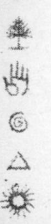

Anita tells us, 'I'm not as angry and selfish as I used to be' following her treatment for glandular fever. When Janie was ill with polycystic ovarian syndrome she told us that she was affected physically, emotionally and spiritually. She is now so much better that she feels she has 'got her life back'. When we become ill we can be affected on all of these different levels.

An acupuncture practitioner doesn't necessarily need to treat 'named' diseases. If you want treatment and are unsure of whether you can be helped by it, ring a reputable acupuncturist and describe your symptoms. She will then tell you if she thinks acupuncture will be of benefit. Of course the only way of really knowing if treatment can help you is by having it and experiencing the results!

WHY DO WE BECOME ILL?

When I was young, my mother would often say things like, 'Don't go out with wet hair, you'll catch a chill', or 'Don't sit on the hot radiators or you'll get piles'. At other times she would tell me, 'Put your slippers on dear', or 'Don't sit on the damp grass', or when I'd played happily in the rain, 'Change out of those damp clothes, dear'.

All of these warnings fell on deaf ears and I definitely forgot about them when I became an adult and didn't have to do as I was told anymore. That is, until I learned about Chinese medicine …

When I studied Chinese medicine I discovered the importance of these 'old wives tales'. They now became 'golden rules'.

I busily started letting my own patients know about them so that they could learn to look after themselves and be protected against the elements of wind, cold, damp, heat and dryness. There were also some other sayings that I realized I could have taken more seriously when I was younger. Some were about our lifestyle such as, 'It's important to have at least one hot meal a day', or 'The hours of sleep before midnight are twice as good as those after', or 'All work and no play makes Jack a dull boy'. Other sayings were about how we look after ourselves emotionally. The Chinese are very strong on these ones and have

proverbs like, 'Laugh three times a day to live longer', or 'A
soft temper is the root of a long life.'

Over time I realized that all cultures had certain 'health rules' which were passed down from generation to generation and which people adhered to. With the coming of modern technology and modern ways of thinking many of these have been lost. Chinese medicine has not forgotten the essence of these guidelines. In this chapter we will learn more about them and what we can do to remain healthy.

Let's find out more from some of the patients we talked to in the last chapter. This time we want to know what they think caused them to become ill.

WHY WE BECOME ILL

Janie, the acupuncture student who had polycystic ovaries says: 'I was born prematurely after dad accidentally locked mum's fingers in a car door. I think it affected my constitution. I was ill throughout my childhood and I was always going off sick with colds. Looking back though I got really ill after I studied too hard and at the same time went on a strict diet.'

For Rose it was more recent. She noted: 'I think I got progressively tireder. I had too much to deal with at work.' Marion's problem was also more recent in onset. She says: 'I always had a slight tendency to get worried but I was never this bad, going on the nursing course really set it off.' Stress is a common cause of illness. Paul noticed: 'It was the stress of my job, managing a laundry was very frustrating at times.' Some people like Edna don't know why they get a symptom: 'I just don't know where it came from. It appeared overnight.'

Patients have their own set of very individual circumstances which lead to them becoming ill and deciding to have acupuncture treatment.

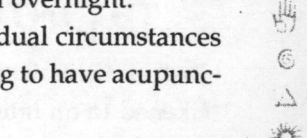

THE IMPORTANCE OF KNOWING ABOUT THE CAUSES OF DISEASE

The more we know about why illnesses arise the better we can prevent them. For instance, if a patient knows that she gets headaches when she is tense at work, she might think twice about getting involved in stressful situations which could bring them on.

We do not have to know the cause of the illness in order to become healthy again – Edna never knew the cause of her frozen shoulder and yet it was cured in a remarkably short space of time. Sometimes, however, it can be helpful to know what the cause was.

THE MAJOR CAUSES OF DISEASE

The Chinese understand there to be three general areas from which disease arises. They call these the Internal, the External and Miscellaneous causes of disease.

The Internal causes of disease come from inside us and are to do with our emotions. The External causes of disease are climatic conditions – the kind of things we were warned about in 'old wives tales'. The Miscellaneous causes of disease are sometimes called 'Lifestyle' causes of disease. They include constitutional factors and lifestyle issues such as diet, exercise, work and rest. In this chapter we will be looking at the Internal and External causes of disease. We will be finding out more about the 'Lifestyle' causes later.

THE INTERNAL CAUSES OF DISEASE

Just as there is an external climate so our emotions can be likened to an internal 'climate'. The Internal causes of disease are anger, grief, fear and shock, worry and over-thinking, and joy.

Even as far back as 2,000 years ago the Chinese understood that our emotional state is a major factor in our ability to remain healthy. Thankfully the link between our emotions and our health has once more been accepted and many people now observe the connection with interest.

It is normal and healthy to express our emotions in certain situations. If we are physically threatened then we naturally feel afraid. If we are badly let down then we will normally feel angry. When the situation has been rectified, for example, the threat is removed or the person who let us down has apologized, then we can move on in life rather than becoming stuck in these feelings.

Sometimes emotions are not so easily resolved. It may be that they are never expressed properly or their expression becomes prolonged and is unresolved. In this case they can become a cause of disease.

HOW OUR EMOTIONS CAN MAKE US ILL

The roots of an Internal cause of disease are often established at a very early age – some people say we have an inherited predisposition to them. A baby has no control over its emotions and will howl with rage if frustrated, feel frightened if threatened, or feel sad if left for a period. A child's emotional state changes rapidly and in most cases she will pass through her feelings and move on to other states as her circumstances alter.

Over time, however, if that child frequently has the experience of feeling frustrated, frightened or sad, a chronic emotional pattern will develop which can weaken her energy. These patterns develop into repetitive emotional states in our adult life. Some people have difficulty with expressing their anger,

others feel anxious and frightened easily and others worry incessantly or often feel joyless and sad for no good reason.

To understand them better we will look at each of these emotions in turn and find out more about how they influence our health.

ANGER

The Chinese say that anger most often affects the Liver. Anger can be anything from resentment, irritability and frustration to extreme rage. It can also lead to depression when it is not expressed.

The Chinese say that anger makes Qi (see page 32) rise and in Chinese medicine it is certainly often associated with headaches. Research at the Saint Louis University Medical Centre in the USA confirms this connection. In a study of 139 people with chronic headaches it was found that those who did not air their frustrations reported more severe symptoms than those who did.

Another study of 63 men with high blood pressure conducted at the University of Wales in Cardiff, found that those who had lessons in anger control coupled with relaxation therapy, had a significant drop in blood pressure. For a long time people have been urged to relax to reduce high blood pressure but the research suggests that curbing the temper is more important. Your acupuncturist will agree. High blood pressure is often associated with anger and the Liver.

Many women feel angry when they are premenstrual. This is also often associated with the Liver. One of my patients describes being pre-menstrual:

'Before my period I used to get so angry that I felt as if I could explode. Every little thing got to me. I'd shout at the children and

then feel awful because I knew they were keeping out of my way.
Then as soon as my period came I felt better.'

The recognition of premenstrual syndrome is relatively new in the West. The Chinese have understood and successfully dealt with it for many hundreds of years. With our increasingly stressful lifestyles in Western society it is far more prevalent now than at any time in our history and Chinese medicine holds a key to its treatment.

GRIEF

Grief is another emotion which can have a strong effect on our health. Grief is a sorrow, a regret, sadness, a sense of remorse or a sense of loss. Grief affects the Lung and we sob when we release our grief.

In the United Kingdom many people keep a 'stiff upper lip' and find it difficult to express their true feelings when someone dies or goes away. One patient expressed the sorrow that he felt as a child:

'I think the illness started when my father left. I remember think-
ing that I shouldn't show my mum that I minded and must be
strong and look after her. Really I felt empty inside.'

This patient never expressed his feelings until later on in life.

Sometimes an unexpressed loss is cleared by acupuncture treatment. One patient told me, 'After my first treatment I cried for the whole day, I realized it was the grief I didn't express when my mother died'.

Grief takes many forms. Some people feel a loss, not because someone has died or gone away but because they haven't achieved what they wanted to in life – what they have lost is a dream but they may still feel just as bereft. *Any* loss can be devastating and a cause of illness.

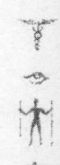

Fear or fright can also be devastating and many people feel it constantly. Fear can be a positive way to help us to be cautious. At the other extreme it can also disable us because of imagined catastrophes that could occur.

One patient who originally came to treatment for his shoulder problem describes his fear:

'Most of my symptoms were caused by fear, I used to have terrible panic attacks and had difficulty sleeping – it was the fear of the fear which was the worst thing and acupuncture helped to ease it.'

Another patient describes what happens when he gets frightened:

'When I'm frightened I breathe more rapidly. My stomach feels tense and I can't concentrate at all. I can be lying in the bath relaxing and reading and see the dark passage out of the corner of my eye and that sets me off. Once a light bulb blew when I put it in and it brought on a panic attack.'

Fear and fright affect the Kidneys. Fright can also affect the Heart. At the other end of the spectrum are situations where people feel no fear although they are in danger. A recent newspaper article describes a skydiver who plunged to his death. His son said:

'Dad loved to take a risk but hated to put his trust in anyone else. Parachuting was his greatest love – he got a real buzz from it and loved to live on the edge.'

This 47-year-old man had predicted that he would die young but still could not resist the lure of danger.

Most examples of feeling no fear are of course not as extreme as this one. Fear or the lack of it can *both* later cause ill health. When we are afraid or do dangerous things, adrenalin is pumped around the body and the resulting tension strains our organs.

Although over-thinking is not, strictly speaking, an emotion, it is still an Internal cause of disease. Worry and over-thinking affect our Spleen and Stomach energy and can include too much studying, obsessive thinking or continually working over something in our mind.

One patient I spoke to had lost 42 pounds in weight in ten weeks before she had acupuncture treatment. She was unable to eat and kept being sick. She tells us why she became ill:

'I think my illness started from the stress of a skin cancer operation. I worried inside and didn't let it out and I also carried other problems. I had reached rock bottom.'

Another patient is typical of some people who worry, 'I'm feeling much better and stronger than I was but I'm now worried about what will happen next – it's all going too well!'

For some people worry gnaws at them even when there is nothing to be concerned about. Here, a teacher tells us how she was affected by obsessive thoughts:

'I got worked up when I got a pain in my breast. The doctor reassured me but I kept thinking it was cancer. I started to feel sick and I'd keep thinking of a friend whose husband had recently died of cancer. I tried to put it out of my mind but I couldn't. It would turn over and over in my head. I couldn't stop thinking that something was really wrong with me.'

She had acupuncture treatment and in time the obsessive thoughts went away. When I saw her two years later she told me:

'I've stayed a lot stronger and have put on weight. I've also coped with two deaths. I very occasionally get a slight twinge in my breast but I don't worry about cancer any more.'

Few patients come to an acupuncturist complaining of being too joyful!

Most commonly people swing from feeling up to feeling down. This patient describes her experience:

'When I'm up I'm really 'high' – isn't life wonderful. Now I'm despondent and frustrated as I don't really understand why I'm down. I feel miserable and I yell at the kids all the time. I find it hard to get out of this miserable state.'

Joy in the context of ill health is not contentment and satisfaction but a more unsettled feeling which could sometimes be described as 'over-stimulation'. Too much joy affects the heart.

Many of us dream of winning the lottery. We might ask ourselves 'How would I really cope?' One sudden burst of euphoria has been known to cause a heart attack and certainly seems to lead to the opposite emotion of joylessness later on. Family break-ups, greed and sadness can often follow on the tail of this sudden joy. As Lao Tse, an old Chinese sage, once said, 'To have enough is happiness. To have more than enough is harmful.'

As acupuncturists, we are perhaps more likely to see patients with the opposite problem – a lack of joy in their life. Here a student says:

'I can get upset for a whole day when someone at college says something hurtful or if I feel I've said something I shouldn't. I feel quite miserable as I don't get on with people as well as I used to.'

This student had acupuncture treatment and as he began to feel better, found he was less vulnerable and could hence get on with other people more easily. He had found greater happiness in his life and this will be important to his future health.

ILLNESSES WHICH MIGHT MANIFEST FROM AN INTERNAL CAUSE OF DISEASE

Almost any illness can result from an Internal cause of disease. Although an emotional cause is frequently rooted in our earliest childhood, illness often doesn't manifest until much later on. Certain conditions such as irritable bowel syndrome, stomach ulcers, insomnia and some headaches are known to be exacerbated by our emotional state but many other diseases also have an Internal cause at their root. The imbalances which come from an Internal cause can affect our bodies or our emotions depending on our current circumstances, constitution and lifestyle.

THE EXTERNAL CAUSES OF DISEASE

The Internal and External causes of disease are often connected. If someone has been weakened by an Internal cause of disease such as sadness or grief, they might then be more susceptible to an External cause.

The External causes of disease come from climatic conditions. These are Wind, Cold, Damp, Heat and Dryness. We will talk about each of these in turn.

WIND

One of my patients described having a common cold. This is a good example of what the Chinese call an invasion of Wind-Cold:

*'I felt fine the day before. In the middle of the night I woke up with
a sore throat and knew I was in for an infection. The next day I
felt terrible. My nose was running, my jaw ached, my eyes hurt,
and I felt extremely tired and shivery. Two days later all my*

symptoms had gone during the day, yet I still woke up coughing at night. It was five days before it went completely.'

What the Chinese call Wind in the body closely matches what they observe in the environment. Wind is something that arises suddenly and goes through many rapid changes. It is often located on the outside of the body and moves in an upward direction. My patient's cold had all of these qualities. She also felt very shivery with her cold as Cold was mixed with the Wind affecting her body.

My patient, like many other people, didn't know exactly why she 'caught', or as the Chinese would say, was 'invaded' by the Wind and Cold. It didn't matter. To have the symptoms of Wind was enough to make a diagnosis.

If she had taken more notice of the old wives tales, however, she might have taken better care of herself and avoided getting ill. Some useful 'golden rules' are: wrap up against cold weather; don't allow yourself to sit in draughty places; beware of changes in temperature – such as moving from a warm environment to a cooler outside temperature; keep your neck covered in windy weather; and don't go out with wet hair.

Other symptoms that the Chinese might describe as arising from Wind may be joint pains which move from place to place, symptoms that come and go such as skin problems or twitches, and symptoms that make us shake or move such as epilepsy or strokes. The climatic factors that can make us ill can combine. In this patient's case the Wind combined with Cold.

COLD

The Chinese describe Cold as something that stops movement and warmth and makes our tissues contract. Pain results from this contraction. A friend's description of wintry weather explains this well:

'I used to feel the cold badly when I was young and I hated it. It wasn't so much feeling chilly that got to me it was more the awful pain in my hands and feet that I disliked. I sometimes even felt it in my ears or my nose.'

Cold contracts the body and, in the case of my friend, the peripheral circulation. Chilblains are one of the most obvious results of extreme cold. They are caused by a narrowing of the blood vessels just below the skin. Cold can also get into our tendons which will cause our joints to become painful, white and contracted.

Other symptoms can be caused by eating too much cold food or drinking too many iced drinks. Our stomach can react by contracting and creating stomach pains or by an inability to digest food. Chronic diarrhoea can also result from eating too much cold food, as can period pains or no periods at all. The advice to eat at least one hot meal a day is very wise.

Another frequent cause of bowel or period problems is Cold caught in the lower abdomen. Avoid sitting on stone steps and other cold places and wear adequate warm underclothes to prevent this from happening.

DAMP

Damp can be caught in the lower abdomen too. It is a very common cause of problems for many people in Great Britain and other countries which are wet or humid. When I teach students about Damp everyone believes that where they come from is the dampest area in Britain!

We don't have to live in a damp area to be injured by Damp. Living in a damp house, staying by or on water, remaining in wet clothes or even doing what the old wives warned us about – sitting on damp grass – can all affect us if we are vulnerable.

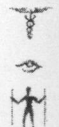

26 Some people are more susceptible to the Damp than others. When I asked one patient how she felt in a damp environment she replied, 'Heavy, thick, sluggish and stiff'. Unlike Wind which comes and goes quickly, Damp is said to be 'sticky and lingering' and is therefore hard to clear.

Feeling stuffy in the chest, bloated in the stomach or abdomen, heavy in the head or lacking in concentration or energy are all symptoms which can be attributed to Damp. In the lower part of the body it can cause bowel problems, fluid retention, discharges or a heavy feeling in the legs. Damp will often create a desire to lie down. One of my patients who has Damp has a saying, 'Why stand if you can sit, why sit if you can lie down?'

HEAT

When we are cold, heat is of course very comforting and soothing. If we are already hot, however, heat can make us extremely restless and be very distracting. When Heat disturbs us it moves upwards to our heads and can make us irritable – 'hot-headed' is an apt term used for people who are hot and bothered and angry.

Sunstroke is the most obvious example of how we might be affected by external Heat. People who work in a laundry or a hot kitchen may also be prone to Heat conditions, as will people who already have a slight tendency to feel hot. Heat can show itself in one area only, such as a red hot painful joint. It may also be all over the body in the form of hot flushes. Heat can also combine with Damp causing infectious or very inflamed conditions which are both full of pus and hot. When we have an infection with a high fever we can be said to be affected by a combination of Wind and Heat.

Sometimes Wind, Damp or Cold, trapped in the body for a long time, can start generating Heat. One good example of this

is cold painful joints suddenly becoming inflamed and
extremely hot.

DRYNESS

This is so rare in England that it is almost non-existent. It is a different story in China. When I went on my first trip to China one of my friends on the trip became ill. She describes her symptoms:

> 'I remember stepping outside in Beijing and breathing in. I had the extraordinary feeling of the cold and dryness going through my nose and deep into my lungs. A few days later it turned into an infection. It was unlike anything I'd experienced before. I had a feeling of incredible dryness in my lungs and an aching feeling in my chest. I had a hacking cough but no matter how much I coughed I just couldn't produce anything.'

She was experiencing an 'attack' of Dryness. For most of us symptoms of Dryness are likely to come from either central heating or during aeroplane flights. Dryness can create any 'dry' symptoms but will often cause a dry nose, throat, lungs or dry skin. A small bowl of water placed in a room is a way of easing a dry atmosphere, especially if it is caused by central heating.

HOW THESE CLIMATIC INFLUENCES 'INVADE' THE BODY

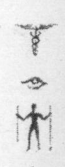

Under normal circumstances most of us can 'brave the elements' with ease and will not be adversely affected by them. There are two common situations when climatic factors can have a detrimental effect. The first is when we are already weakened or susceptible to climatic conditions and the second is if the climatic influence is so extreme that we can't resist it.

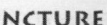

If we feel the cold easily we will be more susceptible to 'Cold' conditions, whereas if we are of a hotter constitution we will be more easily affected by Heat. Some people feel damp weather more than others and they often have weakened 'Spleen' energy. More is written about the Spleen in Chapter 4.

Sub-zero temperatures, a tropical climate or severely humid weather can take their toll on even the healthiest people. One patient who originated from near Newcastle, describes how the elements affected her as a child:

> *'I had rheumatism every winter from the age of 7 to 16 years. I couldn't pick up a pen to write or play with my friends as I could hardly walk. I lived on the North-East coast of England where the winds were vicious, cold, damp and horrible. At the age of 16 I spent three weeks in the Alps where we had solid hot, dry sunshine. I suppose it dried me out. That was the first winter when I didn't have rheumatism. After that I moved to the South of England and didn't go back to the North East. I never had it again.'*

This patient was lucky, the climatic condition that affected her was 'dried out' naturally by the sun. Sometimes a condition won't clear by itself. Acupuncture can then be very helpful.

HOW TREATMENT CAN CLEAR THESE CLIMATIC CONDITIONS

Treatment can be planned specifically using acupuncture points to clear Wind, Cold, Damp, Heat and Dryness from the body. For instance, many points have the word 'Wind' in their name, 'Wind Pond', 'Wind Gate' and 'Wind Palace' are a few examples. Using these and other points will clear conditions in which a patient has Wind in her system.

Dampness is another example. This can be moved using points on the Spleen Channel of the body. This patient describes how she felt when she had Dampness cleared:

*'At one treatment the needles were put in at the sides of my knees.
I felt as if something was flushed out of my body in a gush. I came
out of treatment with a spring in my step.'*

RESOLVING EMOTIONAL CAUSES

Acupuncture can also strengthen the organs that have become
weakened by Internal causes. As treatment balances the energy,
patients often feel healthier and more able to deal with their
feelings. Patients can feel increased well-being quite quickly
and tell their acupuncturist that they feel better in themselves.
This is a sign that the traumas of the past are starting to heal.
Because Internal problems are sometimes very deep seated
they can take longer to treat than External ones.

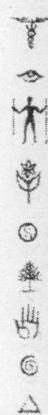

WHAT THEORY IS USED TO MAKE A DIAGNOSIS?

When Edna's frozen shoulder was treated her practitioner unblocked the 'energy pathways' which travelled through that area. Her condition got better very quickly. She said, 'I had the needles in various places. Two or three in the shoulder, as well as some by the thumb and on the side of the hand and one just below the elbow. It was perfectly all right and didn't feel unpleasant at all.'

Anita, who had glandular fever, had 'Damp-Heat' trapped in her energy pathways which was causing her illness. When the Damp and Heat were released her glandular fever went away. 'My acupuncturist put needles in my elbows, the top of my head, the back of my neck and near my knees. They were left in for a while and didn't hurt. They just felt warm and light.'

For Janie it was different. Her complaint lay at the level of her organs rather than in the energy pathways. Treatment strengthened the functioning of her Kidneys and Spleen. She was still treated at points along these energy lines, however, and this in turn affected her organs. She said, 'The needles were all left in and were used on my legs, arms and torso. It was like being plugged into the energy supply.'

In this chapter we will be discussing what we mean by these energy pathways. We will also look at other fascinating parts of the theory of Chinese medicine such Yin and Yang, the functions of the organs, the substances and how the organs are coupled together in 'Elements' which interact with each other.

THE ENERGY PATHWAYS

We know that blood circulates throughout our bodies and that our nervous system gives off impulses. Even if we don't know exactly how a nerve is stimulated or in what way the blood circulates it doesn't matter. As long as we see that we have red stuff inside us called blood and feel movement and sensation from our nerves, then we know that they must exist.

It takes one more short step for us to embrace the concept that we have an energy circulation too. The idea that there are invisible pathways called 'channels' or 'meridians' flowing throughout our bodies has been an integral part of the theory of Chinese medicine for many thousands of years. Fortunately, like us, the Chinese didn't worry too much about proving their existence. That people regained their health when they were treated at key points along these channels was convincing enough for them.

We are now able to measure a difference in skin resistance on the areas where acupuncture points lie. Scientists have also discovered that important substances called 'endorphins' are released when an acupuncture treatment is given. These endorphins are natural painkillers. Pain is only one of the many conditions acupuncture can help and soon we can expect scientists to find other physiological effects which result from acupuncture treatment.

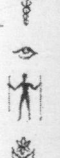

THE ENERGY WHICH FLOWS THROUGH THE PATHWAYS

The energy flowing through these pathways is known as Qi. Qi is less dense than matter so we can't see it. It is nevertheless essential to our well being. Qi is originally made from clean air combining with the food we eat. This mixture then goes through several refining processes before it becomes the Qi that moves through our channels.

The vibrant activity of Qi moves, warms, transforms and protects everything in our bodies. The fact that our blood circulates, that our limbs can move, that our Stomach digests food and our hair grows is because we have Qi. Our Qi revitalizes us. Without it we would be dead. The Qi in the channels connects to and nourishes our organs.

THE ORGANS AND THEIR PATHWAYS

We can compare the channels and organs to the landscape around us. If we had a bird's eye view of any country the first thing we might notice could be the roads. Some of these are large dual carriageways on which cars and lorries can move from place to place. Other smaller roads give people access to more remote areas. The roads are similar to the network of channels which travel throughout the body.

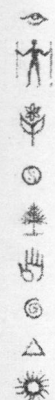

The cities and towns can be compared to the organs of the body. Often a road is named after the town it leads to. In the same way, the channels are named after the organs they join up with. Roads are vital links that bring supplies into the cities and towns.

Sometimes roads become blocked. Most commonly nowadays this is due to traffic jams but it can also be because of an accident, a fallen tree or even snowdrifts in winter. There might also be a food shortage and nothing available to reach the cities or outposts. In both of these cases the residents become desperate when they don't have the provisions they need.

If provisions are cut off for a long time worse problems occur and even looting and violence can result. Similarly, when the channels in the body become deficient or blocked the organs are starved of vital energy. If this continues for a long period, sickness may manifest physically, mentally or spiritually. A problem only affecting the energy pathways is called a 'channel problem' in Chinese medicine.

Sometimes problems in urban areas are not due to bad access by roads but because there is unrest or pollution in the towns and cities themselves. The organs of the body can be affected in much the same way. Rather than being weakened by lack of nourishment from the channels, they can be influenced directly by bad diet, pollution, injuries or emotional problems. In this case the cause of an illness is called an 'organ problem'.

THE CONNECTION BETWEEN THE CHANNELS AND ORGANS

We have just compared the channels to roads and the organs to towns and cities and we know that illness originates when either the channel or the organ is blocked or depleted.

The twelve main channels and organs are all connected. The Heart channel which has a pathway travelling down the arm is joined to the Heart itself. The Small Intestine channel which moves from the little finger across the shoulder blade and up to the face, has a branch which connects it to the Small Intestine organ. Likewise, the Stomach channel is attached to the Stomach organ and the Gallbladder channel is connected to the Gallbladder organ.

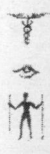

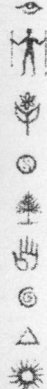

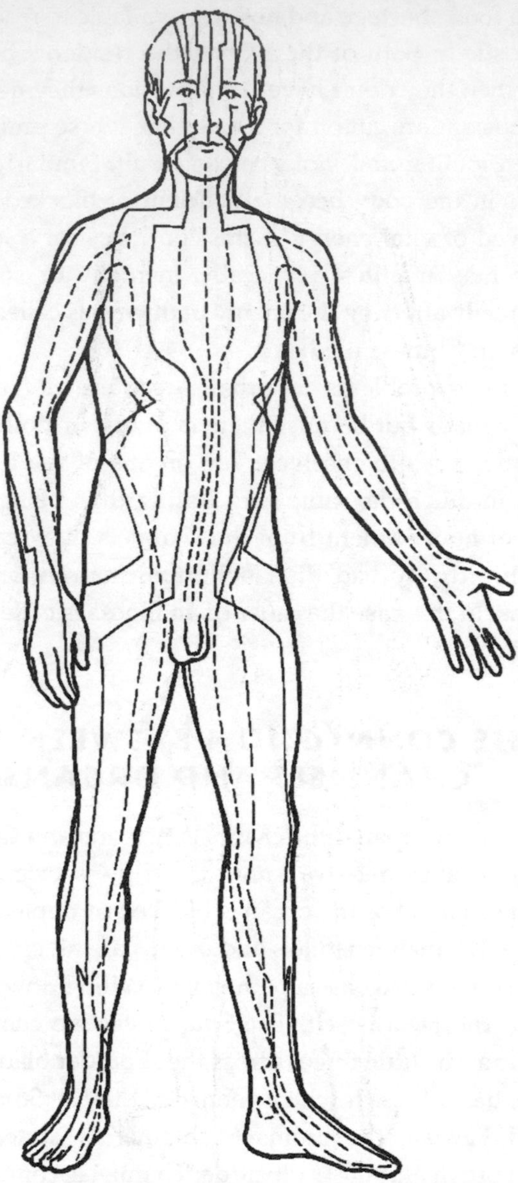

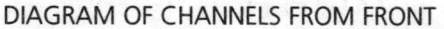

DIAGRAM OF CHANNELS FROM FRONT

PRINCIPLES OF ACUPUNCTURE

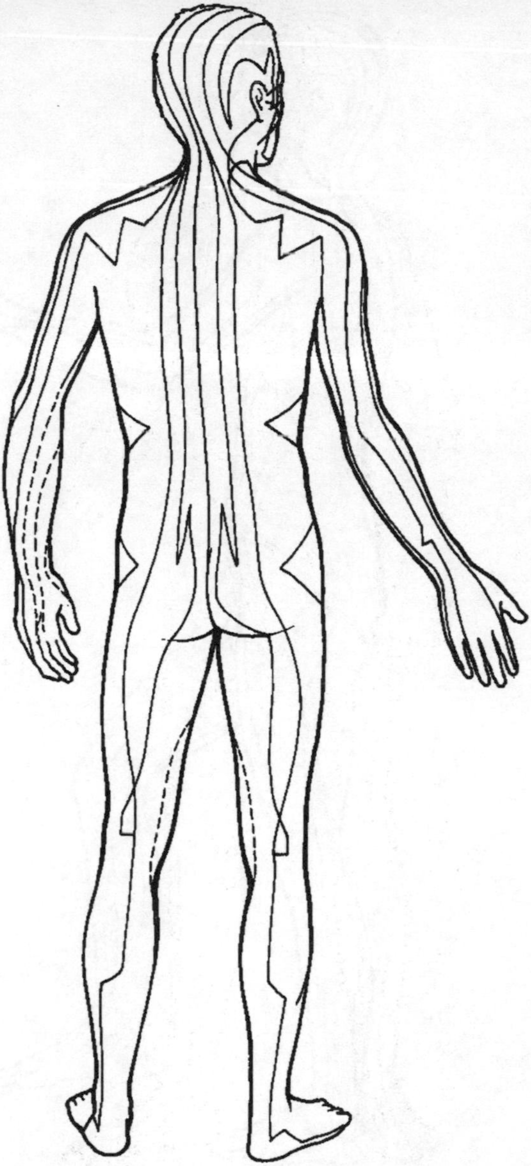

DIAGRAM OF CHANNELS FROM BACK

PRINCIPLES OF ACUPUNCTURE

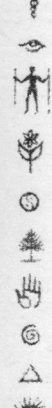

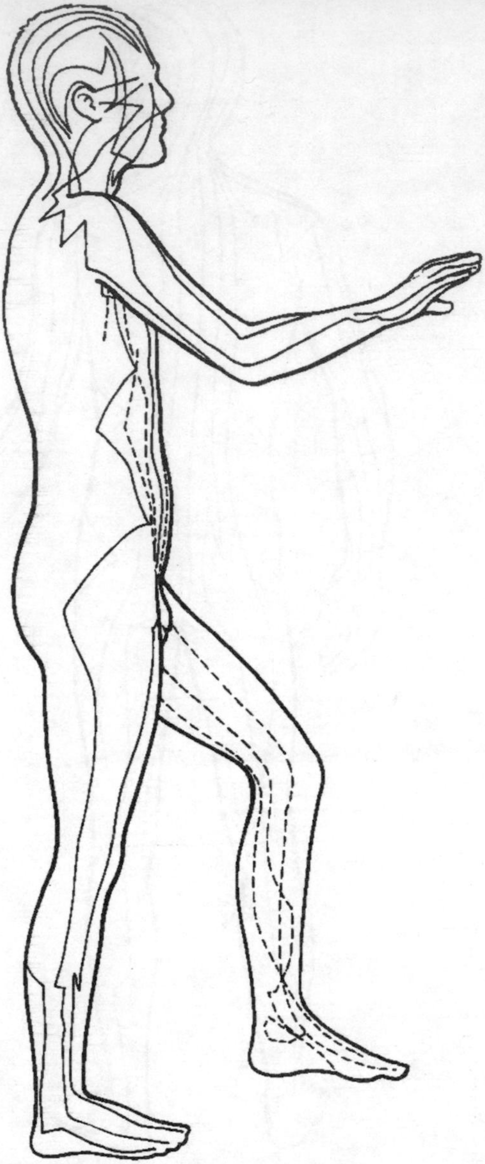

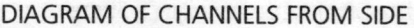

DIAGRAM OF CHANNELS FROM SIDE

The twelve meridians and organs are also paired together. Thus the Stomach is connected with the Spleen, the Gallbladder with the Liver and the Heart and Small Intestines are joined together. The other paired organs are the Kidneys with the Bladder, the Lung with the Large Intestine and the Pericardium with a function known as the Triple Burner. Of these pairs one of the organs is a predominantly 'Yin' organ and the other predominantly 'Yang'.

YIN AND YANG

The Chinese describe every interaction in the universe in terms of Yin and Yang. They are eternal opposites. For example, light and dark, up and down, outside and inside and expansion and contraction are all opposing qualities of Yang and Yin.

There is more to them than this, however. Let us consider light and darkness to illustrate this. Yin and Yang are dependent on each other – we know that without darkness there would be no light and vice versa. They are also in a constant state of flux – both absorb each other and transform into the other. At the height of midday there is maximum light – which is Yang. Around midnight the opposite is true and there is maximum darkness – which is Yin. As the day changes the amounts of light and darkness vary.

As dawn breaks the darkness begins to transform into light. We could also say that the light is 'absorbing' the darkness. The day gradually becomes brighter and more Yang as it progresses. Later as the evening draws in, the day becomes darker and more Yin. Daytime begins to transform into night or we could say that the night-time is 'consuming' or absorbing the daylight.

Yin and Yang have four important qualities:

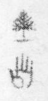

1 They are opposite to each other.
2 They are dependent on each other.
3 They absorb or consume each other.
4 They transform into each other.

Everything in the universe can be described in terms of Yin and Yang but it is important to realize that Yin and Yang are relative to each other. A day is only one small part of the whole year which also has Yin and Yang qualities. For instance, during the year the summer, which is brighter and hotter, is more Yang and the winter, which is colder and darker, is more Yin in quality. When spring arises, the Yin of winter declines and in autumn the Yin is reappearing as the Yang of the summer recedes.

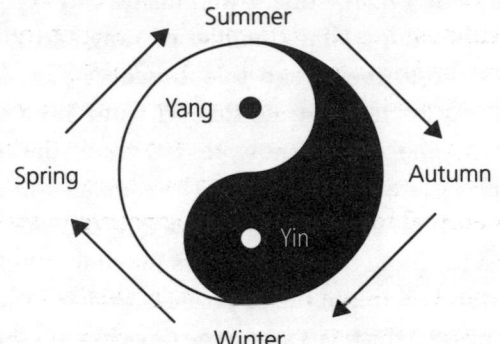

THE SEASONS IN RELATION TO YIN AND YANG

THE IMPORTANCE OF YIN AND YANG TO AN ACUPUNCTURIST

Just as the universe has its own dynamic balance of Yin and Yang, so correspondingly does each individual. In order to remain healthy we need to live in harmony with Yin and Yang in nature.

During the day which is more Yang we are naturally more active. At night, our energy withdraws inside us and becomes more Yin so that we can close down and sleep. If we wish to remain active when we should be sleeping it might indicate that our Yin energy is depleted. When our Yin is strengthened with treatment we become more settled.

On the other hand, if we continually sleep and feel lethargic during the daytime this might indicate that our Yang is deficient. There is not enough expansive and active energy to get us moving. Strengthening our Yang energy in this case can restore our health. Janie who had polycystic ovarian syndrome is an example – her Kidneys and Spleen were both deficient in Yang energy. As a result she found it hard to get up in the mornings and described it as 'like swimming to the surface of a sea of treacle'. Treatment has strengthened her Yang energy, allowing her to feeling bright and lively in the mornings.

Yin and Yang are reflected in the way we live during the seasons and even the cycle of our lives. We are naturally more active and outgoing when it is hot and sunny in the summer whilst it is normal to withdraw and conserve ourselves in the winter.

At the beginning of our lives we are normally very Yang. We move from being energetic children to active adults. Later in life we naturally become more Yin and may wish to slow down. It is very common in the West for people to ignore any signs of ageing. We are encouraged to fight nature rather than work with it. As a result, many people work too hard when they might be resting. This can cause them to become deficient in their Yin energy later in life.

This is especially true of women who at the time of the menopause become hotter, dryer and sometimes more restless – all signs of the Yin energy becoming depleted. It is interesting to note that hot flushes are less common in China, where

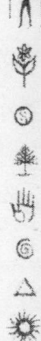

women are more aware of their Yin nature in the latter part of their life, than in the West.

When an acupuncturist examines a patient she will look at how the qualities of Yin and Yang interact and how treatment can bring about a better balance between them. The practitioner might consider the patient's general condition and ask herself, 'Is this patient lethargic or restless, cool or hot or wet or dry?'

The practitioner can also consider Yin and Yang in terms of where the disease is situated in the patient and ask, 'Is this condition deep inside the body or more on the surface?' Or which organs are most involved in the illness, 'Does this patient's condition involve more of the Yin organs or the Yang organs or maybe even both?'

SOME YIN AND YANG QUALITIES

YANG	YIN
Heat	Cold
Light	Darkness
Rising	Descending
Exterior	Interior
Expansion	Contraction
Above	Below
Head	Body
Back	Front

THE DIFFERENCE BETWEEN YIN ORGANS AND YANG ORGANS

The Yin organs are the Heart, Spleen, Lung, Kidney, Liver and Pericardium. The Yang organs are the Small Intestine, Stomach, Large Intestine, Bladder, Gallbladder and Triple Burner.

Yin organs are 'storage' organs and lie deep inside the body. They are responsible for regulating and storing all the body's vital substances before they are used in the body. The Yang organs can be called 'workshop' organs and lie nearer to the surface of the body. They are responsible for receiving, separating, distributing and excreting all the vital substances.

Yin and Yang organs work together. If the Yang organs don't transform the vital substances there is nothing for the Yin organs to store. On the other hand, if the Yin organs can't store these substances there is no point in the Yang organs transforming them.

WHAT THE CHINESE MEAN BY AN 'ORGAN'

When the Chinese describe an organ they are speaking not only of the physical organ but also of some wider functions as well. We will discuss the Yin organs in the greatest detail. They are deeper in the body and have more functions than the Yang organs.

Each Yin organ has i) a main function which is described in relation to one of the 'vital substances' which we will hear about next, ii) an important spiritual function, and iii) an associated sense organ. We will now look at each of these in turn.

THE MAIN FUNCTIONS OF THE ORGANS

The main functions of the organs are all associated with certain 'vital substances'. These substances are the basic constituents of a human being. The energy pathways could be described as the anatomy of Chinese medicine whilst the functioning of the organs and substances could be called the physiology.

There are five main substances. The first is *Qi* which we have already mentioned. The others are, *Blood*, *Shen* or *Mind-Spirit*,

42 *Jing* or *Essence* and *Body fluids*. The Shen or Mind-Spirit is the most rarefied of these and the Body Fluids the most substantial.

The Yin organs have an important role in the storage of the substances. These are their main functions.

1 The Heart and Pericardium 'govern' the Blood and 'house' the Shen.
2 The Spleen transforms and moves Qi and Body Fluids around the body and also 'controls' Blood.
3 The Liver 'stores' Blood and ensures that our Qi flows smoothly around the system.
4 The Kidney stores Jing or essence.
5 The Lung governs breathing in Qi and sending Qi and Body Fluids out to the skin.

THE QI AND ITS RELATIONSHIP TO THE LIVER, LUNG AND SPLEEN

The Qi originates when clean air in the Lung is mixed with the food we eat. The Lungs 'govern' our Qi and our respiration and the Spleen transforms and moves the Qi to every part of the body.

Qi is taken in when we breathe and moves downwards and outwards via the Lung. When the Qi moves downwards the breathing deepens. When it travels outwards it goes to the skin. At the skin the Qi protects us and prevents Wind, Cold, Heat and Damp from causing illnesses such as colds and flus.

The Spleen transforms Qi and transports it around our body. If the Spleen is weak, the Qi can't be moved and we probably feel lethargic. This lack of transportation can also cause our limbs to lack nourishment and become weak or our digestive function to become impaired. Treatment on the Spleen can strengthen our energy and restore our vitality.

Rose who came for treatment to keep herself well had become very tired before she had treatment. This was because her Qi had become very deficient. She told me, 'I used to sleep heavily on Saturdays and Sundays I was so tired. I think it was a progressive tiredness and towards the end of term I went to bed earlier and earlier.' Tonifying Rose's Qi restored the balance of her energy so that she regained her vitality.

The Liver is also connected with the Qi and ensures that it is flowing smoothly and evenly throughout our system. Our emotions are the main cause of disruption to this flow. Try clenching your fists, tightening your shoulders, tensing your chest, holding in the muscles of your abdomen and tensing your neck and jaw. It is hard to imagine Qi flowing easily when we do that isn't it?

Many of us hold our bodies in a permanent state of tension because we are frustrated, irritable, angry or not expressing negative emotions. By doing this we prevent our Liver Qi from flowing. If the Liver Qi is blocked in this way the resulting symptoms might range from premenstrual tension or headaches to digestive disorders, gynaecological problems or depression. Treatment on the Liver can smooth out the flow of Qi and make us feel better. Paul who talked to us in Chapter 2 had headaches due to a Liver problem. He described himself as 'Less sparky, aggressive and demanding' since having treatment.

This is how another patient feels when her Liver Qi is treated: *'I notice a change from the seat upwards. It's as if I'm on a plank of wood gently sliding into warm water. It starts at my feet and travels up my body. It's like lying in the shade and the sun comes up. A warm relaxed feeling washes over me.'*

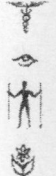

THE BLOOD AND ITS RELATIONSHIP TO THE HEART, LIVER AND SPLEEN

Blood travels not only in our blood vessels but also in our channels. Four organs have a function connected with the 'Blood'. The Liver 'stores' the Blood, the Heart and Pericardium 'govern' the Blood and the Spleen 'controls' the Blood. The organs and their functions in relation to Blood are explained slightly differently in Chinese medicine than in Western physiology.

Blood is 'stored' in the Liver and nourishes and moisturises our whole system. When we are resting the Blood stays in the Liver. Then when we move around the Liver ensures that the Blood reaches every part of the body and nurtures it. If Blood is deficient we might get symptoms due to lack of nourishment such as dry eyes, cramps, pins and needles, flaky nails, scanty periods or dry skin. We might also feel lightheaded when we stand up. This is because there is not enough Blood reaching our head when we move suddenly.

The Blood can also become stuck. This can cause extreme pain. If the Liver Blood is affected it can result in women having excruciatingly painful periods.

The Spleen 'controls' the blood and keeps it in the Blood vessels. If the Spleen is weak the Blood will 'leak' from the Blood vessels which may cause bleeding symptoms such as menstrual bleeding, bruising or blood in the urine or stools.

Finally, the Heart 'governs' the Blood, that is, makes sure it is circulated to every part of the body. If this function is weak we may have poor circulation and cold hands and feet. There must also be sufficient Blood for the Heart to 'house the Shen'.

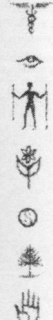

The Shen can loosely be translated as 'Mind-Spirit' and is best described by its actions. First, it helps us to think clearly and to be mentally focused on our activities. Secondly, it allows us to sleep soundly without disturbance. Finally, it gives us the ability to be conscious. This is consciousness both in a sense of having insight into ourselves as well as being conscious rather than unconscious. When our Shen is disturbed it can result in sleep problems, anxiety, jumpiness and a poor memory.

You may remember Marion who was treated for her anxiety about writing essays for a nursing course. Much of her treatment was centred around 'Calming the Shen of her Heart'. Treatment allowed her to think more clearly, remain calmer, sleep better and become less anxious.

Karen who had breast lumps removed also needed her Shen treated. In her case her relationship had broken up around the time she became ill and this had resulted in her Shen becoming disturbed. Treatment allowed her to cope better with her situation and to feel more positive about herself.

In order for the Shen to be settled the Blood of the Heart must be strong as well. The Shen also interacts with the Kidneys and the Kidney 'Jing' or Essence.

JING AND HOW IT IS ASSOCIATED WITH THE KIDNEYS

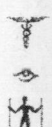

Have you ever wondered why some people get ill easily whilst other lucky people seem to be able to eat anything, stay up all night and generally abuse their bodies without any apparent health problems?

The difference is largely to do with the 'Jing' which creates our constitutional strength. If it is strong then we will have lots of energy and develop normally. If it is weak this won't happen. The total amount of Jing we have is formed when we are conceived and is stored in the Kidney. It has an overall effect on our health. As we go through life we slowly use it up.

Janie who we discussed earlier had slightly deficient Jing – hence she became ill at an early age. She thought being born prematurely must have affected her constitution. Edna on the other hand had a very strong constitution. She describes herself as 'tough'. At the age of 74 she said of her illness, 'I'd always been tough. I hadn't had anything like that before and didn't expect it.'

Maturation from puberty to old age is a natural process that takes place automatically if we have sufficient Jing. Some children are born with weak Jing. They may have symptoms of delayed growth, late onset of their periods, bedwetting, or problems with their bones. When these problems are severe they may be very hard to treat.

We may have plenty of Jing when we are born but use it up too quickly with bad living habits. If this is the case women may have difficulty conceiving or they may suffer repeated miscarriages. It can also lead to an early menopause, back problems or osteoporosis. Losing teeth and hair and a failing memory in old age are all also symptoms of declining Jing.

Most people have a moderate amount of Jing and can avoid these problems if they look after their health fairly well. Those who think they have a super strong constitution should beware however. Bad living habits take their toll in the end and a healthy lifestyle now can prevent problems later. Janie has changed her lifestyle considerably since she had treatment. As a result she can expect to keep her new-found vitality and to have a healthy future.

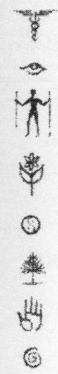

The last substances which we will consider are the Body Fluids which are transported around the body by the Spleen. Some of our fluids are 'light' and lubricate the skin and muscles, others are 'heavier' and moisten areas deeper inside the body such as the joints, spine, brain and bone marrow.

The Fluids must be kept at their correct balance in the body. If our Qi is deficient it can't move the fluids which in turn can congeal and produce 'Damp'. This can cause us to put on weight. This excess weight can be difficult to lose. We can also feel tired, heavy, find it difficult to concentrate and feel cloudy in our head. Treatment can strengthen the Spleen's ability to move fluids. This can clear the Damp and remedy the situation.

The Body Fluids can also become deficient. This can happen if the Stomach is weak and it may result in dehydration. In this case treatment on the Stomach can help to alleviate the problem and bring moisture back to the system.

HOW THESE SUBSTANCES INFLUENCE EACH OTHER

The Qi, Blood, Shen, Jing and Body Fluids are all interlinked. The Qi, Jing and Shen form our basic energy. The Chinese even call a healthy constitution 'Jing-Shen'. The Jing is at the foundation of our Qi and Qi is the basis for our Shen.

The Shen of course cannot be settled unless the Blood is sufficient to house it. The Body Fluids are essential in order to keep the Blood at the correct viscosity.

If one or more of the organs is weak or blocked, the substances they affect will also be influenced. Conversely if the substances are deficient or stagnating this will impact on the organs.

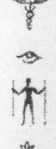

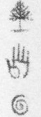

THE MENTAL AND SPIRITUAL
FUNCTIONS OF THE ORGANS

Each organ has a spiritual aspect which will affect a person in certain ways. We have already looked at the Shen or Mind-Spirit and seen how the Heart and Pericardium 'house the Shen'. The Shen can be described both as one of the 'substances' and one of these spiritual functions.

When the Shen is out of balance we can become disturbed and have poor sleep, memory and concentration and extreme restlessness and anxiety. Besides the Shen which is linked to the Heart and Pericardium, the spiritual aspects of the other organs are called the 'Hun', the 'P'o', the 'Yi' and the 'Zhi' (pronounced 'je'). We will go through each in turn.

The spirit of the Liver is the 'Hun' which is sometimes translated as the 'Ethereal Soul'. The Hun has to do with our ability to plan what we do with our lives. When our Liver energy is out of balance we may have difficulty making plans and decisions. As a result we may overplan and try too hard to predict our future needs, or the opposite – be totally unable to make plans. Interestingly the Liver is known to create unpredictable symptoms – making it even more difficult to make plans. As one patient said:

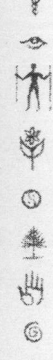

> 'When I'm out of balance I can't make any plans or decisions. As long as there's another possibility I'm not clear what to do. When I'm healthier I have a focused clarity of mind that tells me what to do.'

The next spiritual aspect is to do with the Lungs and is called the 'P'o'. This is often translated as 'Corporeal Soul'. The P'o energizes and animates us. When someone is in high spirits and gets vigorously involved in an activity the Chinese say they have 'P'o Li' which means 'vigorous strength and power'. Patients who have depleted Lung energy are often lacking in energy and vitality and feel there is something missing in their lives. When the Lung is treated this vitality can return.

The 'Yi' is the spiritual aspect of the Spleen. Yi can be translated as thought or 'intention'. Just as the Spleen transforms and transports our physical energy it also moves our thoughts. If the Spleen becomes deficient we may be incapable of 'transforming' our thoughts which can become stuck in our heads making us unable to follow activities through. This patient described to me how she feels when her Spleen is unbalanced:

> 'It's like having a 'mind ache' – the thoughts are going round and round and looping back onto themselves. Then after I've had treatment I feel more clear-headed.'

Finally the 'Zhi' is the spiritual aspect associated with the Kidneys. The Zhi can be translated as our will. Our will or drive in life should be as natural to us as the physical changes that happen as we move from puberty into adulthood and old age – another Kidney function. If the Zhi is weak we will either have no willpower at all or may overcompensate and feel 'driven' to do things. Often people who are driven wish they could stop working but feel unable to do so. As one patient said:

> 'Looking back I realize that I was overdoing it for a long time before I became ill. I was very competitive and under a lot of pressure at work to perform. I hated the stress but didn't know how to stop.'

Treatment on the Kidneys can help a person to slow down and take life as it comes. If a person is at the opposite extreme and has no drive, treatment may help to create more 'get up and go'.

THE SENSE ORGANS AND THEIR ASSOCIATED ORGAN

Besides the spiritual functions each organ has an associated sense organ. In Chinese medicine the Liver is connected to the

eyes, the Kidney with the ear, the Heart with the tongue, the Spleen with the mouth and the Lung with the nose. A malfunction of the organ can affect the corresponding sense organ.

Many eye problems come from an imbalanced Liver. This may manifest in ways such as dry eyes, black spots in front of the eyes, gritty eyes, red sore eyes and other eye conditions. As the Liver energy starts to flow smoothly or the Blood becomes stronger because of treatment, the eye trouble may lessen. Eye problems manifest on all levels and as a patient becomes healthier she may have more 'insight' or 'vision' in her life. Of course this may tie up with other aspects of the Liver such as her ability to plan ahead and 'see' the future and to relax about life so that her Qi can flow smoothly. All aspects of an organ interact.

The tongue is the organ associated with the Heart. Many speech disorders can also be caused by the Heart being out of balance. How many times have you had a word on the tip of your tongue and not been able to remember it? If it happens frequently it can be due to the Heart Shen. Slight Shen disturbance may be affecting the memory which in turn influences our speech. Stuttering is another example. When the Heart is treated this can be a first step to enabling a person who stutters to speak more fluently.

We will briefly go through the other organs. The Kidney is connected to the ear. A weak Kidney can cause symptoms such as tinnitus, dizziness and deafness. The Lung opens into the nose. If we have healthy Lungs our nose will be clear and we can breath easily. If we lose our sense of smell or our nose continually blocks up this may be due to weak Lung energy.

Lastly, the Spleen is connected to the mouth and manifests in the lips. The Spleen allows us to discern the 'five tastes'. Eating too much of one taste such as the sweet taste can imbalance our Spleen as can a dull and unvaried diet. Eating a diet containing a good mixture of different tastes is on the other hand stimulating to the Spleen. Other common symptoms of a deficient Spleen are the loss of our sense of taste, pale lips, sore lips or spots around the mouth.

THE FUNCTIONS OF THE YIN ORGANS

Organ	Main function	Mental/Spiritual function	Sense organ
Heart and Pericardium	Governs Blood	Houses Shen (Mind-Spirit)	Tongue
Liver	Ensures smooth flow of Qi. Stores blood.	Houses Hun (Etheral soul)	Eye
Lung	Governs Qi and breathing	Houses P'o (Corporeal soul)	Nose
Spleen	Transforms and transports Qi and body fluids. Controls blood.	Houses Yi (Thought)	Mouth
Kidney	Stores Jing	Houses Zhi (Will)	Ear

So far we have discussed the different organs and the concepts of Yin and Yang. This chapter wouldn't be complete however without some discussion about one more fundamental concept in Chinese medicine – the Five Elements.

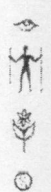

THE FIVE ELEMENTS
AND HOW THEY ARE RELATED

Each of the organs that we have discussed is related to one of Five Elements. The Elements are *Wood, Fire, Earth, Metal* and *Water*. The Liver and Gallbladder are connected to the Wood Element, the Heart and Small Intestine and the Pericardium and Triple Burner to the Fire Element, the Spleen and Stomach to Earth, the Lung and Large Intestine to Metal and the Kidney and Bladder to Water. One of the oldest descriptions of the Five Elements was written as long ago as 1000 BC and it says:

'Water moistens downwards, Fire flares upwards, Wood can be bent and straightened, Metal can be moulded and hardened and Earth permits sowing, growing and reaping.'

The word for Element is *Xing*. This has also been variously translated as a movement, a phase or a moving force. It literally means 'stepping forward with one foot then with the other', suggesting that there is movement and interaction between them.

HOW THE ELEMENTS INTERACT

The Elements connect with each other via the Sheng and Ke cycles shown in the diagram. The Sheng cycle is the route by which the organs nourish each other while they keep each other in check via the Ke cycle. If the energy of one of the Elements becomes imbalanced it will often affect the others.

Paul, who had headaches, was mainly treated on his Liver and Gallbladder which are part of the Wood Element. The emotion associated with the Liver is anger. His Liver Qi had become imbalanced due to the frustration he felt in his job. The Qi rose up to his head causing his headaches. Wood is 'fed' by the

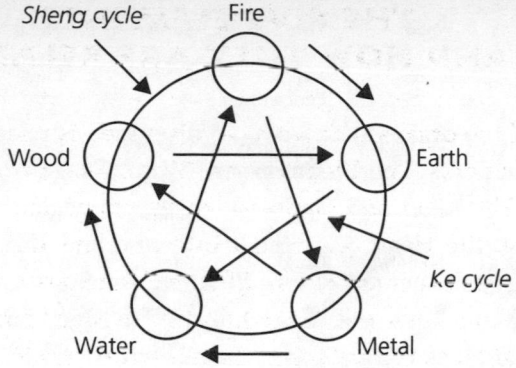

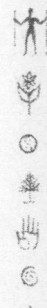

THE FIVE ELEMENTS AND THE SHENG AND KE CYCLES

Water Element. His practitioner told me that she often treated his Kidney energy which is a part of the Water Element and this helped to balance the Liver. On some rare occasions he became nauseous with his headaches – symptoms associated with the Earth Element and the Stomach and Spleen. Treating the Wood affected the Earth via the Ke cycle so the Earth itself very rarely needed treatment.

Treatment on one or more Elements and organs can affect all of the others in a positive way.

When we examine the organs and their related Elements we can understand why they are associated. For example, what better Organ to associate with the Earth – producer of our food – than the Stomach and Spleen, the two main organs of nourishment. The Water Element could only be associated with two organs. They are the ones which transform and excrete fluids in the body – the Bladder and Kidneys. We already know that the Liver is associated with our ability to make plans. 'Wood' energy is associated with all things living and growing. We can move forward and 'grow' as a result of clear plans and decisions formed by a healthy Liver and Gallbladder.

Overleaf is a list of some of the Five Element associations.

	Wood	Fire	Earth	Metal	Water
Yin Organ	Liver	Heart Pericardium	Spleen	Lung	Kidney
Yang Organ	Gall bladder	Small intestine Triple burner	Stomach	Large intestine	Bladder
Colour	Blue-green	Red	Yellow	White	Blue-black
Sound	Shout	Laugh	Sing	Weep	Groan
Emotion	Anger	Joy	Worry / Sympathy	Grief	Fear
Odour	Rancid	Scorched	Fragrant	Rotten	Putrid
Season	Spring	Summer	Late summer	Autumn	Winter
Climate	Wind	Heat	Damp	Dryness	Cold

THE FIVE ELEMENT ASSOCIATIONS

In this chapter we have looked at the channels or 'meridians', the functions of the organs and substances as well as Yin and Yang and the Five Elements. When one or more of the organs or Elements becomes unbalanced our health will be affected in our bodies, minds and spirits to varying degrees.

By diagnosing and treating the imbalances that are at the root of the illness, our health can be restored on all of these levels. If only the symptoms are removed and the main cause is not addressed, the illness will be temporarily alleviated but there will not be a lasting cure.

In the next chapter we will learn how the theory in this chapter is used to create an accurate diagnosis of the patient.

HOW IS A DIAGNOSIS CARRIED OUT?

Acupuncturists are aware that people can be apprehensive when they first come for treatment. One practitioner told me:

'I like the patient to know that I'm really there for them and listening. I'll explain how I'm going to do the diagnosis and that I'll be asking questions so that they know what's happening. I try to put patients at ease and let them know they don't have to go through huge feats of memory in order to answer questions. Then I'll just chat – often about something we have in common or something that's current. I like to make contact before getting on with taking the case history.'

All of the practitioners that I spoke to recognized the importance of good contact with their patients. 'A patient has to feel safe with me before we begin treatment', is the way another colleague put it. Patients value the practitioner-patient relationship too.

Without this rapport it is impossible to carry out a truly holistic diagnosis. Rapport is the vital key which enables a patient to open up and talk to a practitioner. This is especially important if areas in her life have affected her health in the past or now.

As we saw in Chapter 1, people visit an acupuncturist for many different reasons. Sometimes a problem is a physical disorder such as a joint pain or an injury. At other times the condition manifests more mentally or emotionally with depression or anxieties. Whatever the problem a diagnosis is always carried out on the patient before treatment begins.

In this chapter we will follow through the process of a diagnosis and discover what kind of questions a patient is asked. We will also find out what the practitioner is assessing. Later we will see how the theory from the last two chapters is put together to make a complete diagnosis.

WHY THE PRACTITIONER NEEDS TO MAKE A DIAGNOSIS

Treatment is aimed at restoring a patient's health on all levels – physically, mentally and spiritually. The initial diagnosis allows the practitioner to understand how to treat the patient in order to achieve this balance. An acupuncturist understands that health is a very positive state which doesn't only involve the symptoms going away. As a result of treatment the patient can also expect to have more vitality and energy and feel happy to be alive or more contented with life.

During the diagnosis the practitioner will be finding out which organs are at the root of the patient's imbalance, which substances need to be harmonized or strengthened and how the Yin and Yang of the body is balanced. Because each patient is unique, two people with the same symptoms will not have the same diagnosis. Hence a practitioner always carries out a complete diagnosis before commencing treatment. She then decides on treatment based on each patient's individual needs.

THE EXPERIENCE OF
THE INITIAL DIAGNOSIS

Here are some comments from the patients we have already met. Karen who was recovering from breast cancer says:

'My acupuncturist went into my whole life history. I remember talking about my childhood, family life and background. I was the eldest of five children. Now as a probation officer I'm more middle class and feel like a square peg in a round hole. It's stressful keeping a foot in each camp. Going through these issues was extremely helpful.'

Marion was panic stricken when she first went for treatment:

'I was so frightened by my symptoms that if she could help me I didn't mind answering any questions at all. No one had been able to tell me what was happening. I couldn't believe that my acupuncturist understood what was going on.'

Paul who had treatment for headaches told me:

'It was fine. I didn't have any problems with it – I don't think it was needed to cure me but it was nice to have someone to listen to you.'

Rose who had preventative treatment says:

'It was an interesting $1^1/_2$ hours. It was useful in that I was looking at all the aspects of myself and it taught me more about them. When I went home I thought of one or two more things that might be significant.'

Practitioners are as individual as their patients. Some prefer the patients to fill in a questionnaire rather than asking questions verbally. Anita who had treatment for glandular fever told me, 'I had some papers to fill in. I answered the questions and took them with me to the appointment.'

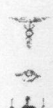

MEETING YOUR PRACTITIONER

The first meeting between the patient and the practitioner is a very important one. The practitioner will greet the patient and take her to a room where she can sit in privacy and talk about her condition. Often the patient trusts the practitioner immediately. Sometimes that confidence grows over time.

The practitioner will also be getting to know the patient. She will be finding out important information which will help her to assess the overall state of the patient's health as well as the cause of the presenting problem.

HOW LONG WILL THE DIAGNOSIS TAKE?

This initial diagnosis will take anything from one to two hours. Some diagnoses are more straightforward than others and some patients have more to talk about so the time varies. The treatments which we will discuss later in the book take less time. These last anything from half to one hour.

WHAT YOUR ACUPUNCTURIST NEEDS TO KNOW TO MAKE A DIAGNOSIS

The four strands of the Traditional Diagnosis are: 'To Ask', 'To Hear', 'To See', and 'To Feel'. The diagnosis has both verbal and non-verbal parts. The acupuncturist asks the patient questions and listens to her and also uses her eyes, sense of touch and surprisingly sometimes her sense of smell, when she carries out the diagnosis.

After initially chatting to the patient, the practitioner will ask the patient many questions. The order in which they are asked varies according to the patient's needs. Here is how one of my colleagues describes questioning the patient during a case history:

> *'I ask patients why they've come and then if they've got any other complaints. We'll talk about the medical history and the different systems such as their sleep and digestion. I'll also ask them what job they do and about their family. I like them to chat about themselves. I think this space to talk is what the patients often don't get at their doctors. I follow up leads when I'm questioning so that I can find a pattern to their condition. I find it's important to get things going so a patient feels comfortable about giving information. Unless they can relax and talk easily I'm not able to bring out what I need to.'*

WHY ASK THESE QUESTIONS?

By finding out about the different bodily systems the practitioner can assess the state of the patient's organs and substances and how healthily she is functioning overall.

Knowing how we sleep, for instance, indicates the state of the Shen or Mind-Spirit and how the Heart Qi is functioning. The Chinese recognize that when we are unable to sleep it is frequently because we are anxious or emotional or sometimes because we are too hot. All of these disturb the Shen. Acupuncture treatment often settles the Shen. Our sleep then improves again.

Our digestion gives the practitioner insight into the functioning of many organs including the Stomach, Spleen, Liver, Gallbladder and Intestines. If we become ill our appetite is often

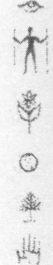

the first thing to suffer, especially if one of these organs is affected. If our appetite declines we stop being able to nourish ourselves properly and further increase our susceptibility to illness. A bloated feeling after eating, heartburn, belching, vomiting or a feeling of nausea can all be indicative of organ imbalances. These will change with treatment as we become healthier.

The practitioner will ask us about other systems such as the bowels, bladder, whether we get excessively thirsty, how much we perspire and menstruation for a woman. She might also question the functioning of different areas of the body such as the joints or the ears, eyes and breathing.

Some questions might not seem to relate to the main complaint at all. Other questions may seem rather strange – for instance, the practitioner may ask about our favourite food, what sort of weather we like or dislike and whether we dream at night. All of these questions are important and will help the acupuncturist to understand our overall state of health.

By finding out the answers to these questions the acupuncturist can not only assess what treatment we need in order to become healthier but also monitor any changes in our condition as we improve.

This is how one patient described being asked questions during the diagnosis:

'We had a one and a half hour session. I thought she'd just be interested in my complaint. In fact she asked me a lot of thorough questions about my background and lifestyle. It was not an inquisition, it was just to get a whole picture. I initially wondered why she wanted to know it. Now I understand the holistic approach.'

'TO SEE'

Throughout the time she is asking questions, the acupuncturist will also be noticing things about the patient. This is the part of the diagnosis called 'to see'. These are the kinds of details that my colleagues observe:

> *'I start by observing the face. I notice its colour and also the expression. I also observe the patient's body language as well as the sparkle in the eyes and the demeanour. I ask myself, "How is their posture?" "Are they bowed in at the chest?" or "Are some parts of the body more developed than others?" '*

This non-verbal diagnosis can be as useful to the practitioner as asking questions. When an organ becomes imbalanced this may show up as a colour on the face. If the Liver Qi is not moving smoothly, for example, this may manifest as a green colour, if we are 'Blood Deficient' we may look a dull pale colour, a weak Spleen may create a slight yellow hue and if we have imbalanced Kidneys we may look dark under the eyes. These colours will all change as treatment progresses.

Body language and posture can also be important. For example, if the Lung or Heart Qi is imbalanced this may be reflected in an underdeveloped chest area. Patients with Damp may have slightly heavy legs if they are women or paunches if they are men. The Kidney Qi affects the spine. When people feel full of vitality they can stand up straight. As the Qi becomes deficient people can no longer hold themselves upright. It is noticeable in some 'less developed' countries that people look more erect in their posture than people in more prosperous countries who often wear out their Kidneys by being overactive.

The acupuncturist may also observe the patient's emotional expression. We have already realized that many illnesses are caused by traumas which began early in life. When we are ill the expression of our feelings can become imbalanced. Some people become more irritable, others find that they can no longer laugh as they used to, while others become more anxious or fearful. Knowing this can help the acupuncturist to pinpoint where the patient's imbalance lies and what treatment

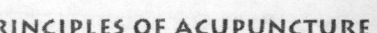

she needs in order to feel better. As patients become healthier their emotions often become more stable. Sometimes patients don't realize that they have felt 'out of sorts' but report after a few treatments, 'I feel better in myself'.

Paul's practitioner did a lot of the diagnosis via observation. She told me:

'Paul's behaviour and voice told me so much that I didn't have to ask certain things at the first visit. Over the following weeks I found out about his past history and he's told me other things.'

'TO FEEL'

The part of the diagnosis called 'to feel' involves examining the patient. One colleague told me:

'If the patient has some physical complaint that needs to be examined I look at it to see where the pain is or what the complaint looks like. I also get an overall picture – are the muscles stiff or is the skin dry or moist? I take the pulse and look at the tongue which are also important. Touch helps a person to relax. If I hold the hand and take the pulses a person often feels more comfortable. One patient told me he'd never been ill in his life before. When I held his hand and he relaxed he remembered he'd had polio as a child.'

Before considering the importance of taking the pulses or looking at the tongue we'll first look at the other parts of the physical examination.

If we have treatment for a painful condition such as a shoulder pain, backache or stomach pains the acupuncturist will want to examine the area. She will palpate the part carefully and by doing so find out how severe the pain is. Dull pain is often caused by deficient Qi whilst severe pain can arise from an excess condition such as Wind, Cold or Damp. If the pain is in a joint she will find out whether or not its movement is

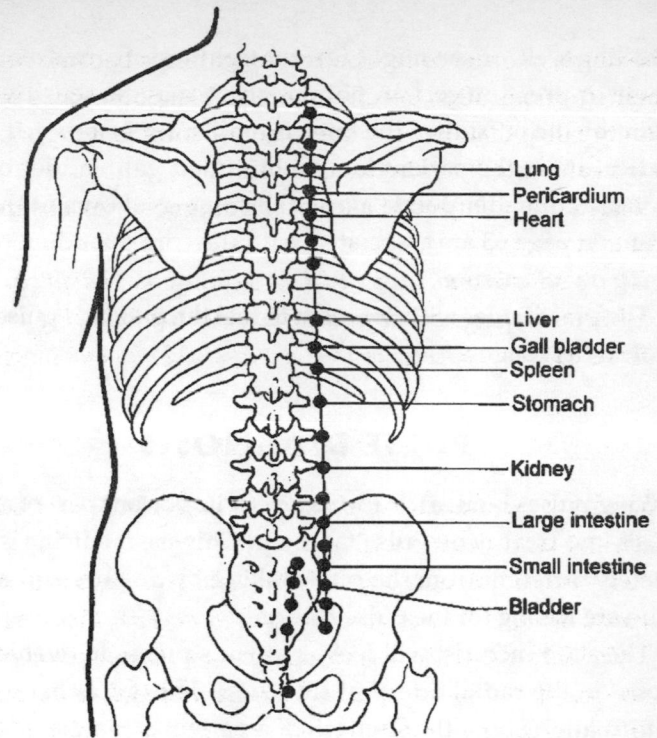

Lung
Pericardium
Heart

Liver
Gall bladder
Spleen

Stomach

Kidney

Large intestine

Small intestine

Bladder

THE BACK SHU POINTS

restricted and whether it is more hot or cold. This is important information both diagnostically and because it will change as the patient makes progress during treatment.

The practitioner will also examine the patient's skin and nails. Problems with the nails are often caused by Liver conditions, especially the Liver being deficient in Blood. Dry skin can have many causes, such as the patient being worn out and deficient in Yin energy, the Lung Qi failing to moisturize the skin or lack of nourishment by the Blood. Greasy skin can often indicate that someone has Damp or mucus in their system.

The practitioner might feel the temperature of different areas of the patient's torso to tell whether the underlying organs are

64 working well, or she might feel for tightness in areas along the spine or press on certain points which may be sensitive. If a point by the outside of the knee is tender, for instance, it could indicate that the patient has an inflamed gallbladder or gall stones and tender points along the spine as shown in the diagram on page 63 are associated with the corresponding organs being out of balance.

The practitioner will also wish to feel the patient's pulses and look at her tongue.

PULSE DIAGNOSIS

Taking pulses is an art. It forms a very important part of a diagnosis and treatment. Pulse taking in Chinese medicine is completely different from the pulse taking by doctors and nurses who are feeling for the pulse rate only.

The acupuncturist will feel a patient's pulses in twelve positions on the radial artery of the wrist. This gives her a lot of information about the strength of a patient's energy as well as the state of her organs. Each pulse position is associated with a different organ as shown on the diagram. The pulses can have many different qualities. Acupuncturists have to practise taking and recording pulses throughout their training in order to become sensitive to the various qualities.

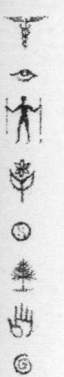

The pulses tend to reflect the internal functioning of the body. Sometimes the pulses are very deep down indicating a deep-seated disease or very near the surface which can show that a condition is on the outside of the body. Pulses can also be strong or weak indicating the strength of a patient's energy or too taut or 'wiry' because the energy is blocked or the patient is tense.

Altogether there are 28 pulse qualities which the acupuncturist might feel. A normal pulse is well rounded, not too strong or weak and normal in its width. Even the healthiest people don't necessarily have 'normal' pulses however. Pulses express our individuality and change according to how we are feeling, the seasons and to some extent the time of day.

Besides being an important diagnostic tool the pulses will alter during an acupuncture treatment and indicate whether we have had enough treatment or if more is required. We will discuss this further in the chapter on treatment.

THE TWELVE PULSE POSITIONS

	Left Wrist		Right Wrist	
	Yang Organ	Yin Organ	Yin Organ	Yang Organ
1st position	Small intestine	Heart	Lung	Large Intestine
2nd position	Gall bladder	Liver	Spleen	Stomach
3rd position	Bladder	Kidney (Yin)	Pericardium	Triple Burner
			Kidney (Yang)	

TONGUE DIAGNOSIS

As one practitioner told me, 'The first time I see a patient I want to know what the tongue is like. It might create more questions and I take the pulses again. Both pulse and tongue are important. I get something to trust from the pulses and tongue.'

Reading the tongue is a very sophisticated method of diagnosis which has been used by practitioners of Chinese medicine for thousands of years.

Our tongues show what is happening inside our bodies. Different areas of the tongue are connected to the different organs (see diagram) and the practitioner will be looking out for any cracks, spots, or different colours in these places.

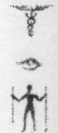
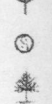

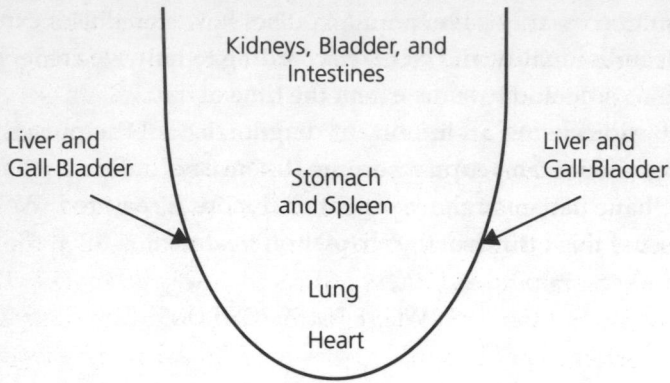

Kidneys, Bladder, and
Intestines

Liver and
Gall-Bladder

Stomach
and Spleen

Liver and
Gall-Bladder

Lung

Heart

THE AREAS OF THE TONGUE RELATED TO THE DIFFERENT ORGANS

The colour of the tongue body is indicative of whether we are hot or cold in different areas. A red tongue indicates a more hot condition and a pale tongue a more cold condition. Cracks or moisture show the state of the body's fluids and movement of the tongue may show the strength of the energy. The coating of the tongue will be especially indicative of the functioning of the stomach as well as revealing whether a condition is more full or deficient.

As treatment progresses the patient's tongue body and coating will change showing that she is becoming healthier.

There is one more significant area of the case history which we haven't yet discussed. This is our family and personal history which covers both more of 'to ask' as well as 'to hear'.

FAMILY AND PERSONAL HISTORY

A famous Chinese doctor in New York puts great emphasis on different phases in our life and how they can affect us. He says that some crucial times in relation to our overall health are:

i) puberty, ii) when we meet a partner and leave home, iii) childbirth, and iv) menopause. These are times when we are changing physically, mentally and spiritually. Having treatment or looking after ourselves during these periods can greatly improve our well being. If we don't care for ourselves at these times then we can become less healthy.

Some patients I see say things like, 'I've never been the same since I went through puberty', or 'I first became ill at the time of my menopause'. Others notice, 'I really blossomed when I had my children', or 'After I got married my health changed for the better'. The acupuncturist needs to know about our history in order to assess these and other factors to do with our overall health now.

An acupuncturist will usually want to know how healthy a patient's parents have been or if there are any illnesses which tend to run in the family. This will give her a clue as to whether there is any constitutional basis to the patient's complaint.

She will also ask the patient about her past history of illnesses. This helps to ascertain whether her problems began before birth, during her childhood or later on in adulthood. For most of us our ailments began at a combination of these times. You may remember, for example, that Janie who had polycystic ovarian syndrome was premature, was often ill with colds as a child, then during her O level exams she over-exercised and ate an unhealthy diet. These all contributed to her illness.

The acupuncturist might ask the patient about any traumas or important events in her life. This 'personal history' enables the practitioner to find out about our present imbalance and its cause. As one acupuncturist says:

> *The personal history gives me clues as to how the patient is now and why they have the symptoms they have. Symptoms don't happen in isolation. People don't just get them without feeling distressed in some way too.'*

68 Emphasis on this part of the diagnosis will differ according to the patient's condition. A patient with a joint problem will have less to say about personal history than one who has other problems which have more emotional causes. Another practitioner says:

'The amount I need to know about a person depends on the problem. If the problem is structural I won't ask a lot about the personal history. I might gather it as I chat to the person while they're having treatment.'

WHAT ELSE MIGHT MY ACUPUNCTURIST NOTICE ABOUT ME?

It was mentioned earlier in this chapter that besides her ears, eyes and touch your acupuncturist might even use her sense of smell. Each of us has our own characteristic body odour. When we were children we may have noticed this more, especially when we had close physical contact with people.

As our energy becomes less balanced our odour will also change. If, for example, we become overheated or our Heart energy becomes unbalanced we may start to exude a slightly scorched odour, and a malfunctioning Spleen can cause us to have a more sweet smell. If our acupuncturist detects these odours it can provide important diagnostic information which can be monitored as we change.

By the time the acupuncturist has gathered together all of the information about the patient she will be ready to form a diagnosis.

MAKING A DIAGNOSIS

As we mentioned earlier in the chapter the acupuncturist will determine many things by interacting with the patient. This includes which organs are constitutionally weak and which have been affected by later events such as emotional traumas, climatic conditions or lifestyle. She will also decide on the balance of Yin and Yang and the interaction of the Substances with the Elements, organs and channels. We'll now look at two of the patients that we discussed in the second chapter and find out more about their diagnosis.

MARION'S DIAGNOSIS

You may remember that Marion came for treatment because she had become anxious and worried about writing essays for her nursing course. Her practitioner told me, 'I was a nurse prior to becoming an acupuncturist and I knew Marion before she had treatment. She was a really capable and confident woman, so much so, that she could take charge of a busy Accident and Emergency department and make it look easy. When she came to me for treatment I was really quite shocked as I hardly recognized her as the same woman. People thought she was nervous but it was more than that and no one was taking her seriously.'

Marion was diagnosed by her practitioner as having a deficiency in her Heart Blood. The Heart Blood keeps the Shen or Mind-Spirit settled in the Heart. Because this was deficient her Shen 'floated' making her feel very unsettled, anxious and unable to sleep or concentrate. The Qi of her Spleen was also deficient. The Spleen is affected by a poor diet and also by constant worrying and these two factors had depleted her.

MARION'S TREATMENT

The first treatment was carried out on the same day as the diagnosis. The practitioner placed a needle in only one point which was on the wrist. This point was to nourish her Heart Blood and settle her Shen. The result was that Marion said, 'I felt a weight lift off my shoulders'. During the following treatments Marion got progressively better. One other area which needed treatment later was her Kidneys.

Her practitioner told me, 'Marion was feeling so much better that she started doing more and more and I think she overdid it.' This brought out an underlying imbalance in her Kidney energy. 'After treating the Kidneys in addition to her Heart Blood she blossomed even more. After one treatment when I treated both her Heart and Kidney energy she told me, 'I felt the energy go up to my head and down to my abdomen. I came awake and had a clearer head.' Her practitioner said of treatment, 'It was wonderful to treat Marion. I felt as if I was on her 'team' and her full participation allowed her treatment to get her better.'

EDNA'S DIAGNOSIS

Edna, you may remember, came for treatment because of pain in her shoulder. Her practitioner told me, 'Edna was in tremendous pain when she first came for treatment. She had already been in pain for five months before coming for acupuncture. Luckily for her she had a good constitution and this had helped her to cope with the pain and helped her to get better quickly.'

Edna told her practitioner where the pain travelled in her shoulder and also answered other questions about her general health such as her sleep and appetite. 'We had a laugh about it', she told me, 'My acupuncturist knew more about me than anyone else.'

Her acupuncturist diagnosed that Edna's problem lay in the energy pathway connected to her Large Intestine. This channel runs along the outside of the arm and over the shoulder and it had become blocked. Treatment was aimed at removing this blockage. Edna's underlying energy also needed strengthening and her practitioner found that she had a weakness in the energy of her chest which affected mainly her Lungs but also her Heart Qi. There is a strong connection between the Lung and Large Intestine in the theory of Chinese Medicine. The underlying deficiency in her Lung energy had probably caused her Large Intestine channel to

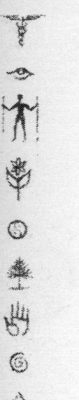

become obstructed in the first place so it was important to both remove the blockage and to strengthen her energy.

Edna had needles in her shoulder but also in her elbow and wrist and she told me, 'The treatment worked well. My shoulder is fine now. During the diagnosis it came out that I'm a bit of an insomniac and I'm doing better with my sleep now as well.'

WHAT DO ACUPUNCTURISTS ENJOY ABOUT DOING A DIAGNOSIS?

There are many aspects of the diagnosis which practitioners enjoy. One practitioner told me:

'I especially like the whole business of someone telling me about themselves so that I know what's going on with them. I can then relate what they say to the theory of Chinese Medicine – sometimes everything fits beautifully into a pattern. Sometimes patients are telling me things for the first time in their lives and as well as giving me information they also find that helpful.'

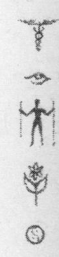

WHEN I HAVE TREATMENT
WHAT WILL IT BE LIKE?

'**B**efore I had treatment all I'd seen was pictures of people with needles sticking out of them. I went in for treatment with an open mind. I just knew it was a very old form of Chinese medicine and that people said it worked but I didn't know why or how.'

People have all sorts of different images of what acupuncture treatment will be like. Here are some other comments from patients:

'I had an absolute aversion to the idea of acupuncture before I had it. I'd tried everything including homoeopathy and herbalism and I then ran my own complementary medicine courses. I liked the acupuncturist who spoke on one of the course days so I decided to have treatment with her. What she said made sense.'

'I'd never considered alternative medicine ever. I'd been brought up very conservatively and acupuncture seemed too way out. I hadn't got a clue what it would be like. The houseman at the hospital said, "Have you considered acupuncture?" I said no. A month later I went for treatment. Now I preach about it to everyone.'

So what will really happen when you are treated? Do the needles hurt? What other kinds of treatments will your practitioner

GOING FOR A TREATMENT

Most patients enjoy having treatment. For example Karen told me, 'It was a joy to go over and be "done". Both the needles and the contact with somebody was important.' Edna said, 'When I went in and my shoulder was pretty bad it was always better afterwards.' Marion's comment was, 'I do enjoy it. It's my time and I know I'm going to have a relaxing hour.'

When a patient goes for treatment the practitioner asks about any improvements that have been made since the last treatment. She will then suggest that the patient sits or lies on a treatment couch while she feels her pulses and looks at her tongue. By doing this she can determine which are the best points to help the patient to progress further.

Having decided on treatment the patient is ready for needles. The acupuncturist will place these in the chosen points. These are often on the limbs although some points may be on other areas of the body.

DO THE NEEDLES HURT?

Most prospective patients find the idea of needles intimidating and acupuncturists are commonly asked whether they hurt. This question is probably best answered by some of our patients.

Marion said, 'I didn't think about them as being needles. I was surprised that they were so small and that there was nothing sharp going into me at all. I do feel a sensation. It's sometimes "nipping", sometimes "warmth" or "like a radiating of something".' Rose told me, 'Many people are frightened of needles.

To me it's just an interesting sensation. I expected them to be left in and twiddled a lot. It was all finer and more delicate than that.' Karen felt the needles occasionally, 'I told my practitioner that she was a bully sometimes. Most needles didn't hurt at all. It was interesting, just a pull. It was fascinating to feel differences in my body in different places. I always felt really positive, whilst with treatment at the hospital I felt negative.' Janie said, 'I don't mind the sensation. It's not a bad feeling. Some points are more powerful than others. It's exciting, if anything, as you're experiencing your energy.'

LEAVING NEEDLES IN

The length of time that the needles are left in varies according to the condition of the patient's energy. If the energy needs to be tonified the needles may be left in for a short time such as 10–15 minutes. Alternatively a needle may be placed in the point and withdrawn almost immediately. A patient with a 'full condition' may need to have the blockage cleared. In this case the needles may be left in for more time. Usually this is up to 20 minutes but it can be longer.

WILL I FEEL THE NEEDLES IF THEY ARE LEFT IN?

If the needles are left in they won't feel uncomfortable. Paul said, 'After the needles are in I then have a quiet time.' Another patient told me, 'Once the needles were in place I never felt them, even if they were left in for 20 minutes.' Most patients feel happy to relax once they are inserted and sometimes even go to sleep.

The acupuncturist will assess how many needles to use according to the patient's condition and the strength of her energy. For example, more needles are usually used for an acute condition than for a chronic one. More are used on someone who has a very strong constitution than on a person who is more fragile. Edna had a very strong constitution. She could have more needles than Marion who felt very fragile when she first came for treatment.

In general two to eight needles will be used per treatment.

DEPTH OF NEEDLES

This will vary according to which point is being used and the size of the patient. The general depth of a needle is from a quarter to half an inch. A point which is on a non-fleshy area of the body such as a toe will penetrate only about one tenth of an inch. On fleshy areas such as the buttock where points are commonly used for hip pain, the needles may go in deeper and be inserted to at least one and a half inches.

THE APPEARANCE OF THE NEEDLES

Many people imagine that acupuncture needles are like the hypodermic ones used for injections. This is not the case. Acupuncture needles are completely different. Hypodermic needles are used to inject substances into the body. In order to do this they have a hollow centre and are relatively thick. In comparison acupuncture needles are extremely fine and solid and nothing is injected through them.

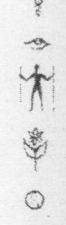

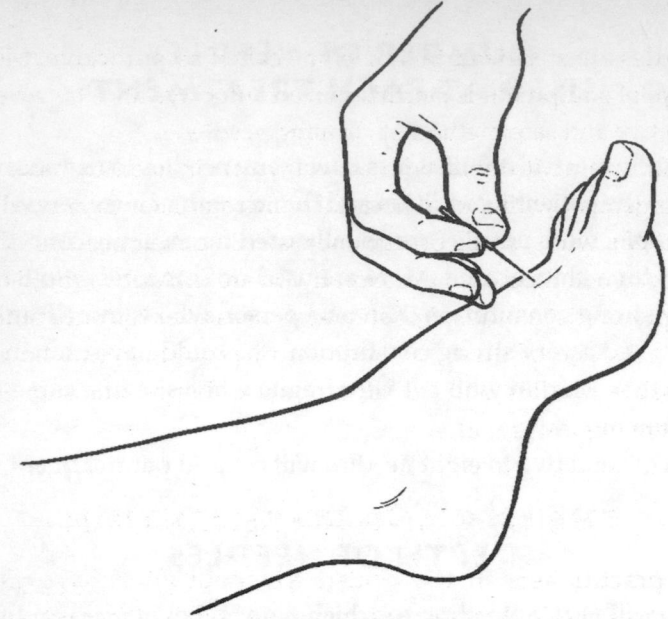

AN ACUPUNCTURE NEEDLE IN THE FOOT

Each acupuncture needle has a coiled handle which makes it easy to hold and of course a very sharp point so that it can pierce the skin easily. The needles are also very flexible so that they cannot break. The length of the needles varies according to which area of the body needs to be treated. Some needles are half an inch, some are an inch long, whilst others are longer.

NEEDLE STERILIZATION

Sterilization is of course another important consideration for all acupuncturists. Most practitioners use disposable needles. These are packed individually, used once and then disposed of.

Some acupuncturists still prefer reusable needles as they are of higher quality than disposable ones. If this is the case the needles are sterilized in a machine called an autoclave. Most hospital equipment is sterilized in an autoclave and it is a very effective and safe method of cleaning needles.

Many practitioners who autoclave their needles have an arrangement with a local hospital which sterilizes their needles for them, whilst some practitioners sterilize their needles in an autoclave in their own practice. If you are in doubt about your acupuncturist's method of sterilization ask her to confirm that she uses one of these methods. Most practitioners who use reusable needles will be happy to use disposable ones if a patient requests them.

THE LAW AND STERILIZATION

All practitioners in the United Kingdom must have their premises checked by an environmental health officer who will also check their method of sterilization. In the United States the Occupational Safety and Health Administration sets requirements for acupuncture premises. A practitioner who is a member of a professional body will also have to prove that they adequately sterilize their needles before being granted membership.

HOW YOUR ACUPUNCTURIST CHOOSES WHERE TO PLACE THE NEEDLES

To decide on where to put the needles the acupuncturist will first choose 'treatment principles' based on the diagnosis.

Marion was diagnosed in the last chapter as having a deficiency of Heart Blood and Spleen Qi. This had resulted in her Shen becoming disturbed. Her treatment principles were to 'nourish Heart Blood', 'tonify Spleen Qi' and 'calm the Shen'. Emphasis

was put on treating her Heart because her constitutional imbalance was in that area. Later on her Kidneys were also treated and a treatment principle to 'nourish Kidney Yin' was added.

Marion's points were chosen based on these treatment principles. Points are chosen for three main reasons: i) they lie on channels connected with the organs which are imbalanced, ii) they have special functions which will enhance the treatment, and iii) the name of the point indicates that the use of that point is appropriate.

Marion needed treatment on her Heart and Spleen organs so points were often used on the Heart and Spleen channels because they feed these organs. She was also treated on some special points on her back which were beneficial for her Blood.

Another point used on Marion was on the lower abdomen. One function of this point is indicated by its name. It is called the 'Sea of Qi' indicating that it is very strengthening to the Qi. Marion also had a point on her wrist treated quite often. This point 'calms the Shen' and is called 'Shen Gate'.

Here Maggie describes one memorable experience of a needle: 'The needle I remember most was on my back. I can remember wanting to just sit with my eyes closed. It was as if I was in another world. It must have been like meditation although I've never done it.' This point was one that had also been used to 'calm the Shen'.

ARE THE SAME POINTS USED AT EVERY TREATMENT?

Whether points are repeated or not depends on the patient and the nature of her condition. Sometimes the points are changed and sometimes they are kept the same. Marion's points were changed quite frequently. This was because as she was progressing and changing internally her needs were shifting. A

point which helped her one week was often no longer appropriate at her next visit.

Edna on the other hand often had the same points treated.
This was because the channel was blocked and treatment gradually cleared the blockage. The same points on her shoulder
and wrist were used at every treatment for a while.

WHAT IS AN ACUPUNCTURE POINT?

Points can be described as small whirlpools of energy. These
whirlpools or 'vortices' are formed where the energy on a channel is disrupted. This is similar to the way whirlpools are
formed when the flow of a river or stream is deflected at a
bend. Points are often found along the pathway where there are
indentations or prominences in the bones or where two bones
meet.

When a needle is placed into an acupuncture point the balance of energy in the patient is changed. Changing this balance
can restore the patient to health.

HOW TREATMENT
RESTORES OUR HEALTH

No one is able to say exactly *how* acupuncture works although
research shows clearly that it does improve our health.

In Chapters 2 and 3 we found out that imbalances in the
energy of our channels or organs will create illness and that
these problems are caused by internal, external or miscellaneous causes of disease. Sometimes the organs and channels
are depleted and at other times they are blocked.

By stimulating the points the flow of the energy is altered.
The energy can then reach a better balance and flow unimped-
ed to the organs. When our energy moves more freely it allows

the functioning of the organs to improve and the channels to unblock. Hence we can regain our health.

THE NUMBER OF POINTS ON THE BODY

Altogether there are approximately 365 points on the main pathways. Some channels have more points than others. There are 67 points on the Bladder channel for instance whilst there are only nine each on the Pericardium and Heart pathways.

The bulk of the points are on the main pathways but there are also some other 'extraordinary' points. For example, the name of one extraordinary point on the neck is translated as 'peaceful sleep' because of its relaxing effects and there are also two points by the knee which are called 'the eyes of the knee'. The eyes of the knee give impressive results in the treatment of many knee problems.

Points can become tender with pressure. One famous Chinese doctor called Sun Si Mao (pronounced Sun See Mee-ow) is reputed to have said: 'If an area is tender then it is an acupuncture point.' Places which feel tender on pressure especially those around joints or painful areas are called 'ah shi' points. Ah shi is translated as 'Oh yes'. When the practitioner presses the right spot the patient says, 'Oh yes that's where it is!'

FINDING POINTS

Not all points can be found by feeling for tenderness. The Chinese have developed a foolproof method by which a practitioner can easily find points.

Using this method the practitioner divides an area of the body up into equal parts. For example, the forearm is divided into twelve equal portions or 'inches'. The Pericardium is a channel which runs up the centre of the forearm. One point on this channel lies at two 'inches' from the wrist crease, another is at three while yet another lies five 'inches' away. By using this method of measurement these points can all be measured accurately and an acupuncturist can always find the points no matter what a person's size or shape.

You may be surprised to hear that needles are not the only form of treatment that an acupuncturist might use. Other treatments that your acupuncturist might use are moxibustion, cupping and cutaneous acupuncture. We'll discuss each of these in turn.

MOXIBUSTION

Moxibustion is the burning of a herb close to or on the body. It is used to warm and nourish our Qi and Blood. 'Moxa' as it is commonly called is made from the leaves of the herb *Artemesia vulgaris latiflora*.

Because the use of needles is so fascinating they often receive more publicity than moxa which is sometimes ignored in the West. Nevertheless the two words that the Chinese use for this therapy are 'Zhen' and 'Jiu'. Zhen means needles and Jiu means moxa. In China needles and moxa have traditionally always been part and parcel of the same treatment.

Most moxa used by acupuncturists in the West is imported from China or Japan. Although the herb mugwort which is commonly found in England is very similar to *Artemesia vulgaris latiflora*, it does not have the same properties.

When the herb is dried it is called moxa 'wool' or moxa 'punk'. Its light brown colour and softness resemble a mixture between wool and cardboard. Its unimpressive appearance is deceptive however. When this brown substance is lit it has an unmistakable aroma which fills the treatment room. It is partly this pungent odour as well as the warmth given off by the burning of the herb which provides its healing effect.

THE USE OF MOXA

Moxa is used for two main reasons. Firstly it warms us up when we have conditions which are particularly 'cold' in their nature. These might vary from a painful joint to a cold lower abdomen or an achy cold lower back. Often a patient describes this pain as 'biting' and she may have already found that the joint, period pains or back problem have benefited from a heat pad or a hot water bottle. In these cases the moxa can produce a strong heat with a penetrating effect. This can 'drive' the cold from the body and over time ease the condition completely.

Secondly moxa can be used to nourish our Qi and Blood. If we feel generally depleted in energy, have a weakness in one or more organs or feel susceptible to the cold weather then moxa can often add to the beneficial effects of the needles. In this case it will gently warm and strengthen our energy.

Janie responded well to moxa because she was deficient in the warming and moving 'Yang' energy of her body and she was diagnosed as being Spleen and Kidney Yang deficient. She said of moxa, 'I love it. My acupuncturist often used a moxa stick – it's wonderful on my back. I could have it all day.'

A moxa stick is one of four main ways that moxa can be used. We'll look at them all.

Moxa can be used as a stick, as small cones, burnt on the end of a needle or burnt in a special 'moxa box'.

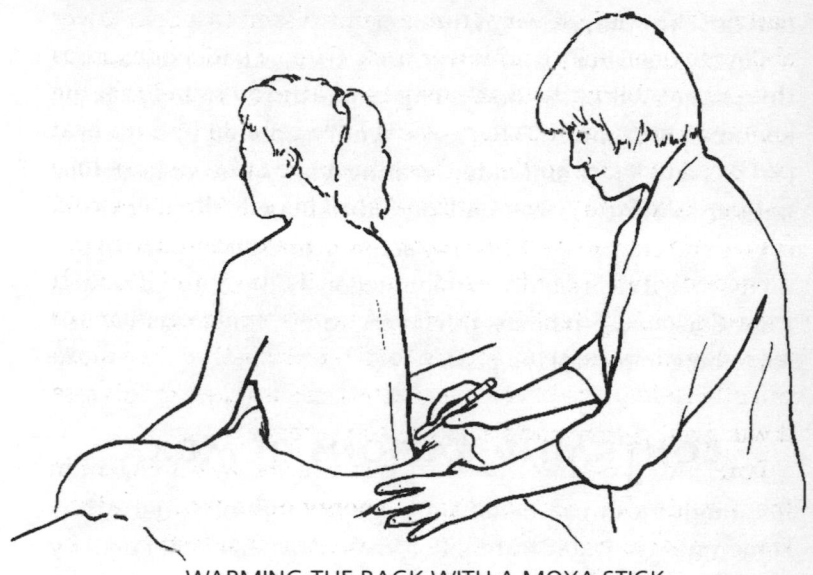

WARMING THE BACK WITH A MOXA STICK

Janie told us that she often had a *moxa stick* used on her back. This stick looks similar to a cigar. After the cigar is lit it is held over a point or moved over an area of the body to nourish and warm it. The lower back, lower abdomen or stomach are common areas where a moxa stick is used although it can also warm a joint or a channel too.

Moxa cones are always used at specific points. A cone is individually lit and allowed to smoulder until the patient feels it become warm. It is then removed. Usually three to seven moxa cones are used on one point although sometimes more are required. This method of treatment is most often used if a patient's energy generally needs to be nourished.

Moxa on a needle is beneficial when deep heat is required at a special point, for instance, when a patient has a painful and cold joint such as a shoulder or hip. The sensation of warmth penetrating deep inside can be very comforting and healing and can clear the cold from the area.

Finally the *moxa box*, like the moxa stick, can be used to heat up a large area of the body. This can also be the lower back, abdomen or stomach. The moxa 'wool' is placed into the special box and left to smoulder creating a large area of heat. One patient told me, 'I once had period pains which were really severe and cramping. When my acupuncturist used a moxa box on the area it cleared the pain miraculously. She then gave me a moxa stick to use at home. It felt very comforting to know I had something to control the pain.'

CONTRAINDICATIONS OF MOXA

Although moxa can benefit a large number of patients it is sometimes contraindicated. For instance, moxa is not usually used if a patient has a hot condition. In this case she might feel very hot, have profuse bleeding such as nose bleeds or heavy periods or have areas of her body which are inflamed or infected. Anita who recovered from glandular fever thanks to having acupuncture treatment never had moxa as she had 'Damp-Heat' trapped in her body. In her case needles were the main form of treatment required.

CUPPING

Cupping originated in China but is still used in many parts of Europe including Turkey, Greece, France and Italy. It removes Wind, Cold or Damp which is trapped in the body and helps Qi and Blood which is 'stuck' or not moving, to flow freely again.

Cupping is often used for joint problems such as swollen, painful or stiff joints and it is also commonly used when we have a common cold and have caught 'Wind-Cold'.

The cups in China are often made from bamboo. Bamboo cups are sometimes used in England too although glass cups are usually preferred. To apply the cups a vacuum is created by placing a lighted taper quickly in and out of the cup which is then placed in position. The patient will not feel any discomfort when this technique is used. As one patient said, 'When I saw the cups I thought they looked a bit strange. When they were actually in place I hardly noticed them, only a slight feeling of suction, that's all.'

If cups are used to clear a common cold the patient is told to wrap up warmly after the cups have been removed. The patient will then sweat and release the Wind and Cold from the body.

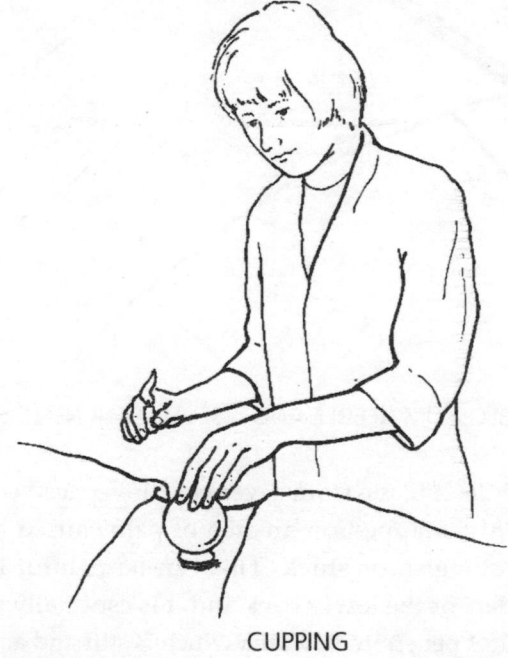

CUPPING

CUTANEOUS NEEDLES

A 'plum blossom needle' and a 'seven-star needle' are the two types of needles used for cutaneous needling. They are made from five or seven stainless steel needles which are inlaid on to a handle. As the word 'cutaneous' suggests these needles hardly penetrate the skin and are lightly tapped on the skin's surface.

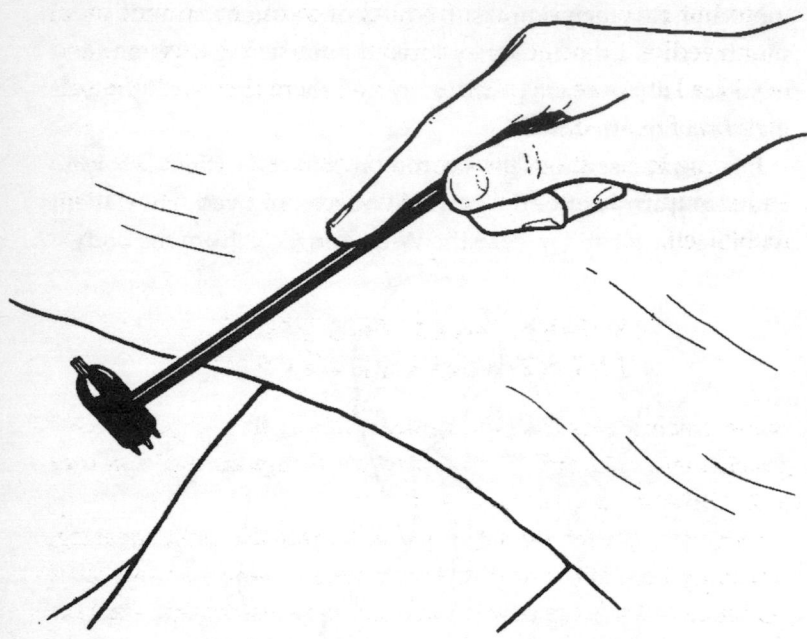

A PLUM BLOSSOM NEEDLE AND A SEVEN-STAR NEEDLE

A *seven-star needle* is made from seven needles spaced equally apart. This is often tapped on an area of pain caused by the energy being sluggish or stuck. This can be painful knees, ankles, shoulders or the lower back and it is especially useful when 'Damp' has penetrated an area which is stiff and achy.

A *plum blossom needle* is slightly different and is made from five needles bundled closely together. It is sometimes called a 'children's needle' because it can be used to tap points on children who are frightened of having needles. We'll hear more about treating children in the next chapter. It can also be used to lightly tap along an energy pathway or a number of points in an area.

Cutaneous needles can be a very effective method of treatment but may be seen less frequently in the treatment room than needles. Some acupuncturists specialize in their use and in China I saw one acupuncture clinic where they were the sole method of treatment.

Having learnt about the common treatments which are used by an acupuncturist, let's go back to find out more about treatment itself.

WHEN WILL THE FIRST TREATMENT BE GIVEN?

Some practitioners treat on the same day as the diagnosis. One practitioner told me, 'I'm keen to get things going.' Another said, 'I always treat at the first session.'

Others may not treat the patient until the next meeting, 'I usually treat at the next session unless someone has an acute problem. If that's the case I do a quick case history and start the treatment immediately.' Another told me, 'Half the time when I first meet a patient and I'm clear about the diagnosis I'll treat. If I want to think about it I don't.'

TIME NEEDED FOR A TREATMENT

This is slightly variable from practitioner to practitioner but it is usually anything from half to one hour.

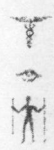

KNOWING THE
TREATMENT HAS WORKED

There are a number of signs that an acupuncturist can detect to let her know that treatment has been effective. At the beginning of treatment the practitioner will feel the twelve pulses which are on the patient's wrist. By feeling them carefully the acupuncturist can discover how the different organs and substances are functioning in the patient. During an acupuncture treatment these pulses will change. The acupuncturist will expect to feel a general improvement in the pulse qualities by the end of treatment indicating that treatment is progressing in a positive way.

The practitioner may also observe small changes in the patient's facial colour or voice tone or she may even notice a renewed sparkle in the patient's eyes. A shine in the eyes is always a good sign. It indicates that the patient's spirit is stronger and more settled and that change is occurring from deep inside the patient. The practitioner may also notice a change in the patient's mood.

CHANGES YOU MAY
FEEL AFTER TREATMENT

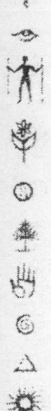

Some patients feel a change immediately after treatment. Others only notice a difference when they look back after a number of sessions and realize that their symptoms have improved. Here is what some patients told me:

Anita said: 'After treatment I was on a high. Buzzing. My body felt as if everything was moving again.' Karen felt an immediate change too. She said: 'I always felt more positive when I came out of treatment. Having chemotherapy and massive contact with the health service was such a nightmare.

Acupuncture helps to deal with the downside of that treatment. I love the feeling afterwards.'

Janie felt a change but in a different way: 'I always used to feel sleepy after a session. The sleep I have afterwards is the most wonderful sleep ever. Now I'm better I don't sleep so much, I'm just very relaxed. It would be nice to snooze but I don't need it.' Paul noticed less immediate change: 'I was not noticeably different straight after treatment.'

Marion told me: 'I felt different after every treatment. Recently I had a slightly fuzzy head for a short time after treatment – like a cap. Sometimes I feel more tired afterwards.' Occasionally a patient feels this slight exacerbation of symptoms before feeling an improvement. This treatment 'reaction' should disappear within twenty four hours.

THE AMOUNT OF TREATMENT YOU NEED

Each patient takes a different length of time to get better. An acute symptom can often be cleared in one to four treatments in quick succession but chronic problems usually take longer. By about the fourth to the sixth treatment the patient will normally have felt some improvement, however, and know that treatment is working.

As a rule of thumb it takes about a month of treatment for every year that the patient has been ill. For some people who have been ill since childhood it may be months or even years before treatment is fully completed; for others only a few sessions will be needed.

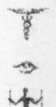

FREQUENCY OF TREATMENT

This also depends on the patient's condition. A patient with a very acute problem might have a few sessions every day or every other day.

Most other patients will start off attending treatments weekly. As their condition improves treatment will be spread out. They may then go for treatment every two weeks, then every three or four weeks. Some patients then prefer to be checked at regular intervals to keep themselves well. Edna still likes to come for treatment occasionally even though her shoulder is now better. Paul on the other hand preferred to stop treatment when the headaches got better.

If an illness stems from some aspect of the patient's lifestyle such as a bad diet, lack of exercise or overwork, then treatment will progress more rapidly if it is changed.

IS THERE ANY REASON WHY A PRACTITIONER MIGHT REFUSE TO GIVE TREATMENT?

Any acupuncturist has the right to refuse to give a patient treatment, but it is rare that this would be the case. A practitioner won't always be sure of how the patient will respond to treatment. If a patient has a chronic and disabling condition such as multiple sclerosis, muscular dystrophy or Parkinson's disease she may tell her what she thinks treatment can achieve. Sometimes, although treatment may not give a complete cure, it can help a patient to feel more comfortable and to cope better with the complaint. How much can be accomplished in these situations is not always easy to assess until a few treatments have been carried out.

If an acupuncturist thinks that treatment will not help a patient she will let her know or recommend another treatment that she thinks might be more beneficial. However, it is important to remember that what an acupuncturist asks herself is, 'Can acupuncture help this person?' rather than, 'Can acupuncture help this illness?' One of the main differences between acupuncture and Western medicine is that the acupuncture practitioner treats people rather than diseases and looks at the whole person.

HOW ARE CHILDREN TREATED WITH ACUPUNCTURE?

In China, many families bring their babies and children for acupuncture if they are ill. When I was doing clinical work in a hospital in China I would often be stunned to see the whole family come in with the child. Families knew how effective the treatment could be and they all wanted to give their support.

Here in the West children's acupuncture is a speciality which is becoming increasingly popular. One mother, Anne, took her one-year-old son David for treatment. Here she tells us about his treatment.

DAVID'S TREATMENT

'I took David for acupuncture treatment because I believed in it. I'd had acupuncture on and off over a long period of time and had even been cured of an acute prolapse of the womb in just one treatment. It had also helped with panic attacks and a number of other symptoms.

'David has quite severe cerebral palsy. It is a spastic form which means he gets quite stiff. Acupuncture treatment didn't cure all of his problems but it helped him tremendously. I once asked a physiotherapist to gauge how severely affected he was on a scale of 1–10. She said if 10 was the worst case she's seen, he was about 8.

'One way in which treatment was stunningly successful was in the treatment of his eyes. He had a squint and eyes which rolled

back. After one particular treatment his eyes came down and could focus. They've never gone back to how they were before and that was four years ago. He has also been helped with his head control and he's surprisingly never developed the chest problems which are usually found in children with cerebral palsy. The medical professionals would often say to me, "Why hasn't he got a bad chest like other cerebral palsy children?" and I'd always say, "It's because of acupuncture."

'*Altogether David was treated for about four years. The treatment didn't help his constipation and although it had some effect on his spasms it didn't clear them either. But I think that having the treatment has made it possible for me to keep him from having the drug treatment which would normally be given to cerebral palsy children. This means that he has been able to develop unusually good cognitive function. He can follow instructions and do school work and I'm pleased that he knows where he is, who he is and will try to do lots of things.*

'*He hasn't had treatment for about eighteen months as it got difficult for me to take him. Now a friend has offered to help out. She saw how much he benefited from the previous treatment and she's offered to take him again – I'm delighted as I'm sure he can get even more improvement and I know it'll be worthwhile.'*

COMMON COMPLAINTS
TREATED IN CHILDREN

David is one of many children who have gained substantial improvements from treatment. Children can have acupuncture for a large variety of conditions.

Children respond really well when treated for acute conditions like colds and flus and other infections such as tonsillitis, mumps and measles. One acupuncturist I spoke to told me, 'Sometimes when a child has a high temperature which

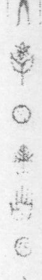

antibiotics can't help, then acupuncture can do the trick.' Acupuncture can also help conditions such as digestive disorders, insomnia, bowel problems, coughs, asthma, bedwetting and some skin conditions.

HOW DO CHILDREN DEAL WITH NEEDLES?

As the same colleague said:

'Using needles on children requires a certain skill on the part of practitioners who will strive to introduce them in a way which doesn't upset the child. The child won't see the needles. Although half an hour might be needed so that the child is relaxed and ready for treatment, the whole process of using the needles will probably take no more than about two or three minutes and the needles are not usually left in.'

In the previous chapter it was mentioned that a 'plum blossom needle' can be used on children who are frightened of needles. This can be an alternative to ordinary needles although it isn't usually necessary. My colleague said, 'Children are usually happy to come back for more treatment and happy when they leave.' David's mother told me, 'David is extremely sensitive to touch and although he has been known to cry with needles, he always knew that it helped afterwards and would look forward to the next treatment.'

CHILDREN'S RESPONSES TO TREATMENT

Children often respond extremely quickly to treatment. Sometimes it is possible to get results in one to two treatments and even if it does take more time a child's energy tends to change much more rapidly than an adult's.

Robin is another child who benefited from acupuncture treatment. He is now 15 years old and he first had acupuncture when he was 13. His mother told me:

'Robin was diagnosed as having asthma when he was $2^1/_2$ years old. He's never been a bad asthmatic but at that age we realized that he was allergic to dog hair and if he caught a cold it would go to his chest. He was prescribed a drug called Bricanyl and later on took a Ventolin inhaler if he needed it.

'At the age of 11 years I took him to a doctor who pushed very hard for giving him Becotide which is a cortisone-based drug. This doctor even went as far as to say that if he didn't have it he would get a heart problem and his growth would be stunted. The doctor wanted him to take this inhaler every day to get it into the system. I refused to give him this treatment and he continued on Ventolin when he needed it.

'I took Robin to an acupuncturist when he was 13 years old. I think it was at exactly the right time and it has had an extremely positive effect. His chest has been so much better and he no longer takes inhalers at all. He initially had three treatments and then had a few boosters later. He had a treatment just before his exams recently. Normally he's a worrier. This time he's coped incredibly well and has been very relaxed. I think that treatment has helped him through them.'

This is what Robin says he experienced from treatment:
'I'm very sporty and always used to feel very tight-chested after distance runs or playing sports. Treatment has allowed me to breathe more freely and I'm now able to do sports without being overwhelmed by them. I can play football 3–4 times a week now with no trouble.'

HOW DOES CHILDREN'S ACUPUNCTURE COMPARE WITH ACUPUNCTURE FOR ADULTS?

Robin's condition was chronic but children can be treated for acute conditions too. Children's illnesses such as infections, chest problems and convulsions often develop more swiftly than adult illnesses and can quickly become more serious. Because of this it is important that children get immediate treatment.

Children's illnesses are often related to digestion. The Chinese say that a child's digestive system is more delicate than an adult's and hence they can only take food which is easily assimilated, such as milk. The digestive system can easily become strained, causing food to accumulate in the system.

Adults and children can both be strongly affected by emotional stresses. For some children these strains can have negative consequences for the rest of their lives. If treatment changes the impact of these stresses it can have a profound effect on the child's future. As one practitioner said:

> 'The difference between treating children and adults is rather like
> the difference between a light lace doily and heavy worsted fabric.
> Children's energy is so light and moves so easily that changes can
> be profound. It's rewarding to put the child's health back to where
> it should be – something has been invested in the child's future,
> in the very weave of the fabric.'

Finally, fewer needles are needed to treat a child than an adult. A young child often needs only two to four needles to have the required effect. The needles are not retained in a child though they sometimes are in an adult.

Treating children is a worthwhile experience for those acupuncturists who specialize in their treatment. As another acupuncturist said, 'What could be more fulfilling than investing in the health of the next generation.'

WHAT OTHER FORMS OF ACUPUNCTURE TREATMENT ARE AVAILABLE?

I was delighted when my cat Minnie had two kittens a number of years ago. She was a good mother and both of them thrived under her care. When they were about eight weeks old I gave one kitten away but decided to keep the other as he would be company for her. For a while she continued to care for Spot until at about twelve weeks she inexplicably rejected him. Spot found the rejection hard to take and tried to follow her around. Minnie's response was to suddenly turn on him and hiss until he went away.

After a while Spot developed diarrhoea. Worse still he became incontinent and was going all over the house. I took Spot to the vet a number of times. After frequent prescriptions he said the only thing left to do was to open him up. Alarm bells rang in my head at the thought of surgery. I decided that alternative measures were required and I would treat him.

For various reasons I decided to treat Spot's Spleen. The Spleen rules over the intestines in Chinese medicine and is also connected with issues to do with a lack of mothering and nurturing. Using only one needle I treated a point on the inside of Spot's foot.

The next day Spot had no diarrhoea for the first time in four weeks. Not only that, he also seemed happier than he had been for a long time and more independent from Minnie. Spot's new-found health continued in spite of Minnie's continued rejection. In the end, I conceded that Minnie was not going to adjust to Spot and I gave him away to a friend. He continued to thrive and became a huge burly tomcat. My friend kept in touch and told me that Spot never had a bowel problem again – thanks to one carefully chosen needle.

For those who think that acupuncture is all in the mind there are many more stories like these that can be told by animal lovers. Veterinary acupuncture is fast becoming very popular. In this chapter we will hear from an acupuncturist who treats animals. We will also find out about a popular method of treating people who are drug dependent and look at some other more unusual methods of treatment such as ear acupuncture, electro-acupuncture and acupuncture anaesthesia.

TREATING ANIMALS WITH ACUPUNCTURE

A colleague who uses acupuncture to treat animals says:

'85 per cent of the animals I treat are dogs. I also treat some cats and the occasional horse. Dogs are very controllable so are easy to treat. Cats are more fidgety but can be good. They co-operate for a shorter time. Horses are easy if the owner is with them and is a good owner.'

DO THE ANIMALS MIND HAVING NEEDLES?

My colleague also said:

'I do the treatment either in a room at the back of the vet's surgery or in a house. It has to be a non-threatening environment. The animal usually spends some minutes sniffing around and exploring

and getting into a relaxed and happy mood. The nurse and I sit with the animal between us and it's important to make sure that it doesn't know it's being restrained. An animal is usually happy and cooperative if treated nicely. Dogs don't feel the needles at all as they have no nerve endings on their skin. Cats can feel them a little bit more and it's slightly more difficult getting their co-operation. Horses become very calm with treatment and I know instantly that the treatment has worked.'

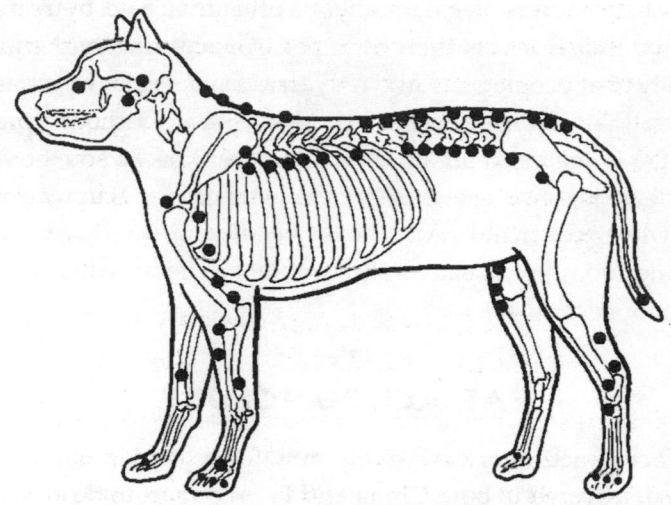

ACUPUNCTURE POINTS ON A DOG

COMMON ILLNESSES ANIMALS CAN BE TREATED FOR

The kinds of illnesses in animals which respond best to acupuncture are arthritic joints to do with old age and normal wear and tear. Intestinal and tummy conditions and backs, as well as problems with mucus can be treated well. As the veterinary acupuncturist says:

'The nice thing about treating animals is that the acupuncture works dramatically. The animals often become brighter and have more energy and the owner frequently says things like, "This is my old Fred again". Animals usually get better – I would say about 90 per cent of the time. So this work is very gratifying to do.'

THE LAW AND TREATING ANIMALS

At one time it was illegal for anyone other than a vet to treat an animal unless it was their own pet. An acupuncturist could legally treat people but could only treat animals in the presence of a vet! The law has now been changed and as long as the practitioner is qualified and the animal has been checked by the vet, it is legal for an acupuncturist to give treatment. If you have a pet who needs treatment, ask your vet. If your veterinary practitioner does not use acupuncture, he or she may know of a practitioner who does.

EAR ACUPUNCTURE

Ear acupuncture is a relatively new form of acupuncture. It was discovered in both China and France at around the same time. In 1956 Dr Paul Nogier, an acupuncturist and neurosurgeon, reported his experiences of ear acupuncture. He was at a congress in Marseille and described using it to treat many conditions. The Chinese were at the same time also finding out about its far-reaching effects.

They both discovered that points on the ear corresponded to different parts of the body. The lobe of the ear, for example, corresponds to areas on the head, the inside of the ear to the internal organs of the body such as the Liver, Spleen, Stomach and Lungs, and the outer ear to the upper and lower limbs.

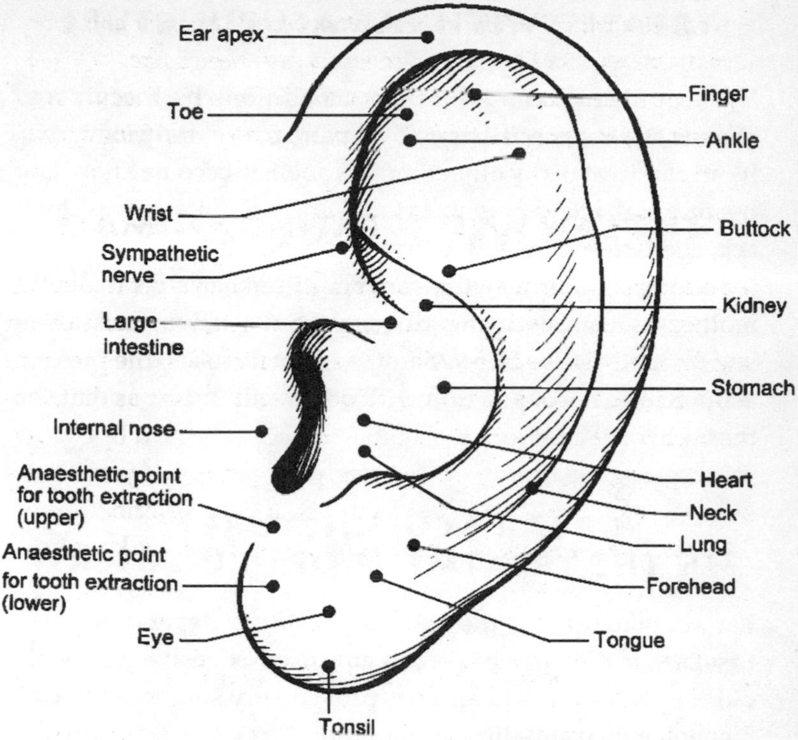

EAR ACUPUNCTURE POINTS

By observing the ear and examining it carefully with a blunt probe, areas of tenderness can be found. These indicate where problems lie in the body. These points can then have needles inserted into them or small seeds attached in order to treat the areas that are imbalanced.

CONDITIONS WHICH ARE EFFECTIVELY TREATED WITH EAR ACUPUNCTURE

Ear acupuncture can treat many conditions both acute and chronic and is especially good for pain, particularly joint pain. It can also treat many other illnesses and has become known for treating high blood pressure as well as conditions such as stomach, chest, intestinal and urinary problems. It can also be helpful during childbirth. In this case points can be used to calm the mother as well as being directed at the pelvis and lower abdomen to stop pain. Many acupuncturists will use ear acupuncture in conjunction with other acupuncture points on the body.

EAR ACUPUNCTURE IN THE TREATMENT OF DRUG USERS

Ear acupuncture for the treatment of drug dependency was first used in the early 1970s. It is now used extensively throughout the Western world and has proved very successful in conjunction with counselling techniques.

An acupuncturist I spoke to ran a drug rehabilitation unit in London for a time. She said:

'In my opinion this treatment is excellent and makes a huge difference. There are five points on the ear that are used to detoxify the body. They help to reduce the pain of withdrawal including such things as vomiting, cramps, sweats and pains in the joints. They also reduce the craving. When people are withdrawing from drugs they are often jumpy, aggressive and agitated. This treatment stimulates the calming "Yin" energy of the body and settles people down. Often people fall asleep during treatment.'

Those withdrawing from drugs have treatment every day if possible. The drug rehabilitation units provide a group situation which is a supportive environment for people coming off drugs.

DRUGS WHICH
RESPOND TO TREATMENT

Ear acupuncture was first used on methadone users. It was then found to be useful for cocaine, crack cocaine, ecstasy, heroin and many other drugs as well as prescription drugs like Valium.

COMING OFF DRUGS

The time it takes to come off drugs varies. Opiates such as heroin can be cleared out of the system in as little as two to three days or up to two weeks. Methadone is much harder and takes longer. Interestingly, cannabis stays in the system for about one month and tranquillizers are the hardest to deal with, taking from twelve to eighteen months to completely disappear from the body.

This form of treatment should be used in combination with good counselling provided by the drug rehabilitation centre. Drug users often start by attending a group where they have ear acupuncture. They might then have one-to-one acupuncture treatment where the acupuncture is directed more towards their individual problems.

STAYING OFF DRUGS

One survey in a hospital in the United States found that 90 per cent of withdrawal symptoms were relieved by the treatment, 90 per cent of patients continued having acupuncture treatment

after coming off the drugs by using the detoxification points, and 60 per cent of patients were still drug free after several months. Tom is an example of one patient who is currently being helped to come off drugs.

TOM'S STORY

Tom has had treatment for only nine weeks and he has already noticed that it has made a difference in many ways. He is 46 years old and is married with two children. This is what he told me:

'I have ear acupuncture four days a week. It is amazingly helpful. In fact I'd now rather have needles than take a pill! Before having treatment I was on 80 mg of methadone as well as diazepam and cannabis. I'm now down to 20 mg of methadone and I've stopped taking the diazepam altogether. I stopped diazepam after the third or fourth ear acupuncture session – I'm very impressed. I still smoke cannabis occasionally.

'I have a long history of drug taking. I started smoking cannabis as a teenager, then joined the army and took Dexidrine and Benzidrine. I left the army in 1970 and went into the music business. From then on it was "sex, drugs and rock and roll" all the way. I was on heroin for 14 to 15 years. It began as an experiment which got out of hand. I went on to methadone as a substitute for heroin and have been on a methadone programme for 18 months.

'Recently I realized that I needed help and that's when I started the ear acupuncture. My wife and I both took drugs and we knew that we couldn't keep taking them now we have the children. We have to clean up our act. Now I'm down to 20 mg of methadone I'll reduce by two mg at a time when I'm ready.

'As well as having ear acupuncture I have normal acupuncture treatment to help me to build up my emotional strength. At the moment my defences are low – I watch Blue Peter and want to burst into tears. If I go in for treatment feeling anxious I feel relaxed and easy afterwards. Acupuncture seems to act as a buffer

for me. It's so interesting that I can have a needle in my toe and it helps me feel better. I've done very well so far and look forward to the day I come off drugs altogether.'

A colleague told me: 'Although it is hard to document how successful this treatment is in the long term, it is known that in terms of abstinence from drugs, whenever acupuncture is introduced to a unit the statistics noticeably improve and the drop-out rate falls from around 70 per cent to 30 per cent.'

The problem of drug abuse is unfortunately on the increase. This treatment is one successful way of assisting patients with the problem. We can hope that it will become progressively more popular in the drug rehabilitation centres and that more research into its efficacy is carried out in the future.)

ELECTRO-ACUPUNCTURE

Electro-acupuncture is frequently combined with ear acupuncture. It is the stimulation of acupuncture points by an electrical current. A small machine which is about five inches long, four inches wide and three inches high is connected to the acupuncture needles via leads which clip onto them. The leads are plugged into output sockets and the stimulation is controlled via dials on the machine. After the machine has been turned on the patient often controls the amount of stimulation going to the needles.

ELECTRO-ACUPUNCTURE VS TRADITIONAL ACUPUNCTURE

Electro-acupuncture is most frequently used when a patient has a 'Full condition' and often when there is a lot of pain. The reason why it is so effective for many of these conditions is that it strongly clears through the channels when there is a blockage.

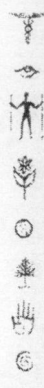

One acupuncturist who frequently uses electro-acupuncture told me:

'I would normally treat a painful condition with ordinary acupuncture treatment first. If the problem wasn't responding I would then use electro-acupuncture. In extreme circumstances, however, I might use it straight away. I also find muscle spasms and circulatory problems respond well to this treatment too and I sometimes use it to calm and relax people.'

SENSATIONS WHICH CAN BE FELT FROM ELECTRO-ACUPUNCTURE

When the needles are initially inserted into the points the sensation will feel the same as in ordinary treatment. The volume of the electrical current is then slowly turned up until the patient feels a slight tingle around the point or along the energy pathway. This sensation is never stronger than is tolerable. The muscles may twitch a little bit but this is always kept to a comfortable level too.

HOW LONG ARE THE NEEDLES LEFT IN?

The needles are left in for as long as the patient needs them. This is usually 20 to 30 minutes. If a condition is extremely painful, for instance a kidney stone is being passed or a gallstone is causing obstruction, then they may be left in for longer.

ELECTRO-ACUPUNCTURE FOR ANAESTHESIA

Acupuncture anaesthesia is carried out using electro-acupuncture and it has been used in China since the 1950s. When I was in China in 1980 I saw two patients successfully having their thyroids removed and one having a heart operation using acupuncture as the sole anaesthetic.

Acupuncture anaesthesia is carried out using the same small electro-acupuncture machine to stimulate the points. The electrical current which stimulates the needles is turned up slightly higher until it comfortably numbs the area which is to be operated on. Ear points or points on channels close to the area to be affected are used.

This form of anaesthesia can be extremely effective for certain conditions, especially those on the upper half of the body. It is an extremely safe anaesthetic for frail or elderly people, entailing less risk and a better recovery time. If it is used more extensively in the future it could help to cut down on the cost of the expensive anaesthetics which are presently used.

We may have a long wait before acupuncture anaesthesia is used on a large scale in most countries. Acupuncturists do not often specialize in this kind of treatment and tend to work in their own private practices rather than in hospitals. There is a growing trend, however, for acupuncturists to work in medical practices. The more acupuncturists there are working in the general medical field the greater chance there is that this treatment will gain in popularity in the future.

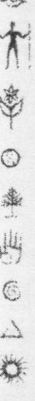

WHAT GUIDELINES CAN I FOLLOW TO HELP ME STAY HEALTHY?

Health is relative. 'Healthy' to some people means that they no longer have the symptom that they came to treatment with: 'My bad knee is better now so I'm all right'. To others 'health' means that they have relief from their symptoms and also generally feel better and more vital in themselves. Most acupuncturists will look for both internal and external changes in a patient's health to assess whether they are better.

Whatever our criteria for 'good health', it is always worthwhile considering how we can best maintain the changes once we have achieved them. Sometimes this involves making adjustments to our lifestyle. We can also have preventative treatment in order to stay healthy. In this chapter we will look at how to remain healthy by having preventative treatment and by adjusting our lifestyles where necessary.

PREVENTATIVE TREATMENT

Rose came for treatment in order to stay well. Edna, Marion, Karen and Janie still have acupuncture in order to remain healthy even though they no longer have the symptoms that brought them to treatment. Paul and Anita stopped having treatment once they felt fit.

When patients like Edna, Marion, Karen and Janie wish to carry on having treatment the acupuncturist will generally be delighted to continue. A patient will then come for treatment every two to three months or at the change of season.

If the patient has no symptoms this doesn't matter. The acupuncturist can still observe the patient's pulses, tongue, facial colour and emotional balance to assess her energy. Treatment can then harmonize any imbalances that have started to occur.

Preventative treatments can be compared to having a regular check-up with the dentist. A periodic visit to the dentist doesn't guarantee that we don't get a bad tooth between check-ups but it can ensure that minor tooth problems are detected before they lead to major ones.

Huang Fu Mi (pronounced Hwang Foo Mee) was a famous doctor who was born in the year 215 AD. He noted the importance of preventative treatment and said that it is the highest form of medicine. He said that treatment is best carried out *before* a disease has manifested.

Ill health often arises after major stresses or changes in our lives. If we are having preventative treatment and further problems do arise we can always go back for more treatment when necessary. Stresses and strains inevitably occur in our lives. Having regular treatment can often help us to deal with them more effectively so that they don't cause major illnesses later on.

Sun Si Miao (pronounced Sun See Mee-ow), born 582 AD, was another famous Chinese doctor. He also talked about preventative treatment and said that many diseases can be cured by regulating our lifestyles. If these lifestyle changes don't work, acupuncture or other forms of Chinese medicine can then be used for treatment. We'll briefly talk about lifestyle and how it can affect us.

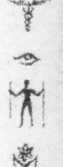

THE IMPORTANCE OF
A HEALTHY LIFESTYLE

An in-depth study has been conducted into the lifestyles of many people in America over the last 30 years. It was carried out at the University of California School of Public Health and identified seven deadly health 'sins' that are likely to lead to an early and painful death. They are:

1 Obesity
2 Physical inactivity
3 Smoking
4 Too much alcohol
5 Sleeping too little or too much
6 Eating irregularly
7 Skipping breakfast.

In the study 7,000 adults were followed from the 1960s to the present day. It was found that these poor habits in combination could *double* the chances of dying prematurely or of developing chronic illnesses.

Although smoking and alcohol were by far the most deadly of the 'sins' it was discovered that even slim, teetotal non-smokers whose only sins were to skip breakfast, eat between meals and sleep irregular hours were far more likely to suffer health problems or to die prematurely than those who led a healthier lifestyle. 'It seems that *regularity* of lifestyle must be health maintaining,' said Dr Breslow, who ran the study.

THE CHINESE AND HEALTH

The Chinese would agree with these findings. Statistics prove that Chinese people generally know more about how to remain healthy than people from other cultures. According to a government survey, in every age group, people of Chinese origin who live in Britain are less likely to suffer from a serious long-term illness than any other race.

The findings of the office of long-term censuses and surveys are that 29 per cent of Chinese pensioners have a serious long-term illness or handicap, compared with 36 per cent of white people and 43 per cent of people of Indian or Pakistani origin.

Lifestyle is important. Eating healthily and regularly, getting enough rest and exercise and protecting ourselves from the elements will help us to remain healthy. Combining this with a calm and happy disposition or 'laughing at least three times a day' as the Chinese say, will ensure a long life.

DIET

Everyone differs in their dietary needs. As a general rule, eating three meals a day at regular times and without eating too late at night will maintain the efficient functioning of the digestive system.

Contrary to some current Western thought, the Chinese say that the Stomach and Spleen tend not to like too much uncooked food or cold food, especially when the weather is cold. Warm cooked food is more easily transformed and digested than cold food. Iced food or drinks straight from the fridge take a great deal of energy to digest and are a definite 'no no'.

Keeping a good balance in the proportions of food we eat is also important. It is best to eat lots of grains and beans and also fruit and vegetables, with smaller amounts of very nutritious foods such as meat, fish, eggs and dairy products. Flesh foods and dairy products are important for our health but are classed as very 'rich' and as such should not be eaten in large quantities.

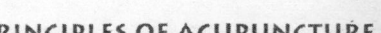

WORK AND REST

Many people push themselves way beyond their natural capacity to work. In China most people will have a rest after lunch before they start working again. A small study in Britain has shown that more accidents take place between 2pm and 4pm than at any other time of the day. Our brains are programmed for sleep not only at night but also after lunch. This makes driving more hazardous and can also have repercussions on the quality of the work that we do.

In England and the United States people often work through their lunch breaks and on into the afternoon – often on a diet of sandwiches and other cold foods. The saying, 'all work and no play makes Jack a dull boy (or Jill a dull girl)' is just as important now as it was in our grandmothers' day!

EXERCISE

Getting a balance between too much and too little exercise will vary from individual to individual, and taking notice of our bodies' needs is very important. Too much exertion can be just as bad for us as not exercising at all and people have been known to overstimulate themselves to the point of collapse because they are obsessed by fitness – on some rare occasions this can be fatal.

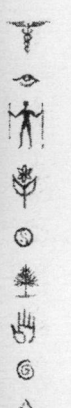

The problems of too little activity are just as bad and studies have found that children are taking one third less exercise than they were in the 1930s. Research at Exeter University in Devon has found that nearly one third of the ten-year-old girls studied and one in five of the boys studied were so inactive that they did not even manage a brisk ten minute walk during the one week in which they were monitored. Because they were taking so little exercise children were eating nearly one third less in

calories than they did 60 years ago and they were more over-
weight!

In these days of increased car use, more television and computer games, children easily miss out on exercise. Activity needs to be encouraged more strenuously to prevent young people establishing habits dangerous for their future.

HOW SOME PATIENTS HAVE CHANGED THEIR LIFESTYLES

Some of the patients we have talked to in the book have noticed the effect of changing their lifestyles. Janie told me:

'I've changed everything. I used to go to bed at 3 am – now I'm always in bed before midnight. Apart from changing what I eat, I now time my last meal for before 7 o'clock in the evening – I used to eat at 10 o'clock. I now always eat breakfast. I used to starve myself, though really I think I was killing myself. I no longer eat fatty food and I've cut out sugar. I also don't over-exercise now. I listen to my body and if I'm tired I don't do it.'

Janie was leading a very irregular lifestyle before she had treatment. Fortunately most of us don't have to make such extreme changes in order to maintain our health. If the task of making changes seems huge then making only small changes bit by bit is the best answer.

Here is what Karen, who had cancer, says about her change in lifestyle:

'I think becoming seriously ill was the greatest crisis in my life. I thought I wasn't going to survive. Life is so different now. I think about it differently and deal with problems better. When I get up I even think about what pleasure I can have today and how my life can be better in quality.'

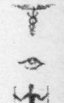

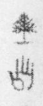

WHERE CAN I GO FOR TREATMENT?

H aving read this book, you may now be thinking about how to find a good acupuncturist. This is how Edna decided to go for treatment.

'I was desperate with my shoulder before I had treatment. I knew a lady who was so ill that her husband had carried her in for treatment and she'd walked out. I spoke to her about treatment and then thought, "I wonder, shall I go?" I did and went in and made an appointment even though I didn't know anything about treatment or how it worked.'

Here is how some of the other patients heard about treatment. Paul said: 'I went for acupuncture as there were no other treatments left – I'd tried everything else! I'd heard about it for many years. Someone at work had gone for something else and gave me my practitioner's name.' Anita read about treatment in a book: 'My mum had gone with a frozen shoulder and brought a book for me. It seemed a natural thing to do anyway. I used to pass the clinic. You go to a doctor or you go to an acupuncturist if you are ill.' Rose found out at a talk: 'I went to a meeting where my acupuncturist gave a talk. I'd felt theoretically in favour and had never tried it, so this was my opportunity.'

Edna, Paul, Anita and Rose all had one thing in common. They had all had an acupuncturist recommended to them or had met the practitioner before having treatment.

Recommendation is by far the best way of finding an acupuncturist. Some towns have many practitioners, others have very few. Too much choice can be as much of a problem as too little. If there are a large number of acupuncturists in your area then you may need to decide which one is best suited to you. If you talk to people who have already had treatment and ask them about their experiences it will help you to decide.

If you can't find anyone who can recommend someone, then ask a practitioner to have a short chat to you about treatment. This will allow you to meet the acupuncturist, ask any questions and see the premises. If you then feel comfortable with the practitioner you can book an appointment.

If you don't know of anyone in your area or if you have doubts about a practitioner's qualifications, you can phone one of the professional acupuncture bodies in your country. Addresses of organizations who will pass on the names of professional bodies in many countries are listed at the end of this book. These societies will gladly tell you who is practising in your area and ensure that you are recommended to an acupuncturist who is well trained.

CHECKING THAT YOUR ACUPUNCTURIST IS WELL QUALIFIED

There are a number of ways for you to check that your acupuncturist is properly qualified. First, make sure that she takes a thorough case history before starting treatment. No practitioner can treat you holistically without making a diagnosis first. A good practitioner will also feel the twelve pulses on your wrist and look at your tongue when she first sees you and at all subsequent treatments.

Find out about her training. Most acupuncturists will have completed a three- or four-year course before qualifying. Some doctors or physiotherapists have done courses which take only a few weekends and are mainly aimed at relieving pain. Practitioners who have taken short courses are *not* well qualified as acupuncturists even if they are first-rate practitioners in their own profession. Some doctors or physiotherapists have completed a full training, so it is worth checking. A poorly qualified practitioner will not be able to achieve the same results with treatment as one who is well trained.

Finally, one of the most important things to notice about your acupuncturist is how you get on with her. Is she interested in you and does she make good rapport? Do you like and trust her? When I talked to patients about treatment it was clear that they placed a high priority on the relationship they had with their acupuncturist.

Marion told me: 'If you build up a relationship you can confide more easily.' Rose agreed: 'I think it's very important that we got on. You have to be comfortable. If you accept how powerful it can be, you have to have real confidence in the person treating you.' Karen added: 'I think how you get on with your practitioner is massively important. Without that relationship, treatment wouldn't be as effective. She was wonderful.'

PREPARATION FOR A TREATMENT

No special preparation is needed before a treatment, although it is best to arrive feeling as well rested and relaxed as possible. Try not to do anything too extreme beforehand such as eating a huge meal, having an excessively hot bath or being strenuously

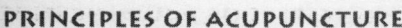

active. If you have had your Liver Qi treated don't drink alcohol after treatment. Your Liver can become very sensitive and small amounts will then have a strong effect.

SHOULD I TELL MY DOCTOR THAT I AM HAVING TREATMENT?

You are not required to tell your doctor that you are having treatment although many people like to let them know. Most doctors, though not all, feel comfortable if their patient is having treatment and in some cases even recommend it. Whether you tell your doctor or not depends on what you are being treated for. If you are taking prescribed drugs then it is best to inform them. The issue of coming off any drugs can then be addressed if necessary.

PRESCRIBED DRUGS AND ACUPUNCTURE TREATMENT

You will not need to come off your drugs in order to have acupuncture treatment. As you become healthier through treatment, however, you may wish to cut down on any drugs you are taking and if possible stop taking them. This depends on the drugs and why you are taking them.

Your acupuncturist is trained to understand the effects of drugs and will advise you on this. If you wish to start reducing your drugs she will often ask you to consult your doctor and withdraw the drugs with the doctor's full support.

Some drugs can be cut down naturally, for example, a patient will stop taking painkillers if she no longer has pain or will gradually cut down on sleeping pills as her sleep improves. Other drugs cannot be withdrawn at all, for instance, some replacement drugs such as insulin for diabetics or vitamin B_{12}

118 for patients with pernicious anaemia. If patients are unable to fully withdraw from some medical drugs, treatment can still help them to improve their health generally and to cope better with their illness.

Having heard about how to find a practitioner we'll hear a few words from Marion:

'I knew I felt better when I could go into the course and no longer wished something would happen to me on the way. It'll soon be my last day at college – I've done all the essays and had my results and I've passed! I'm going back to Accident and Emergency again soon. I went back to see what it was like and I felt really at home. I've felt so different from treatment and I've never reverted back to how I was before.'

I hope this book helps to open more people's minds to the potential benefits of acupuncture and at the same time dispels some of the myths about needles. For those of you who have decided to have treatment, I hope that you are helped in at least as many ways as the patients who have talked to us in this book. We'll have one last comment from a patient:

'I think acupuncture has really changed my life. It's helped me to enjoy life. I was so poorly I thought, "This is how I'll be for the rest of my life". Everything in me was at rock bottom, now I'm a stronger person from it and my whole lifestyle has improved. I'm very grateful.'

USEFUL ADDRESSES

If you wish to find out more about acupuncture you can ring the societies listed below.

UK

British Acupuncture Council, Park House, 206 Latimer Road, London W10 2RE. Telephone 0181 964 0222.

AUSTRALIA

Acupuncture Association of Victoria, 126 Union Road, Surrey Hills, Victoria 3127. Telephone 613 95322480.

Australia Acupuncture Ethics and Standards Organisation, PO Box 84, Merrylands, New South Wales 2160. Telephone 1800 025 334.

Australian Traditional Medicine Society, 120 Blaxland Road, Ryde, New South Wales 2112. Telephone 809 6800.

CANADA

The Canadian Acupuncture Foundation, Suite 302, 7321 Victoria Park Avenue, Markham, Ontario L3R 278.

NEW ZEALAND

New Zealand Register of Acupuncture, PO Box 9950, Wellington 1. Telephone 04 8016400.

USA

Council of Colleges of Acupuncture and Oriental Medicine, 1424 16th Street NW, Suite 501, Washington DC 20036. Telephone 202 265 3370.

National Accreditation Commission for Schools and Colleges of Acupuncture and Oriental Medicine, 1010 Wayne Avenue, Suite 1270, Silver Spring, MD 20910. Telephone 301 608 9680. Fax 301 608 9576.

National Acupuncture and Oriental Medicine Alliance, 1833 North 105th Street, Seattle, Washington DC 98133. Telephone 206 524 3511.

National Commission for the Certification of Acupuncturists, 1424 16th Street, NW, Suite 501, Washington DC 20036. Telephone 202 332 5794.

If you wish to find out more information from the author you can contact her at: The College of Integrated Chinese Medicine, 19 Castle Street, Reading, Berkshire RG1 7SB. Telephone 0118 9508880.

INDEX

abdomen, bloated feeling 26

aches and pains 1–2

acupuncture points 31, 78–81

  on dogs *99*

  ear *101*

acupuncturist, finding 114–18

acute disorders 12, 93, 96, 102

acute infections 2, 93

'ah shi' point 80

anaesthesia, electro-acupuncture for 107

anger 18–19

animals, treatment 97–100

Anita, case history 8–9

Artemisia vulgaris latiflora 81

asthma 94, 95

back Shu points *63*, 64

balance, and disease 80

bedwetting 94

Bladder 40

  paired with Kidneys 37

and Water Element 52, 53–4

blockages 32–3, 47, 64, 74, 79, 106

Blood 41, 47

  organ association 40, 44

Body Fluids 42, 47

  organ association 42, 47

bowel complaints 11, 25, 26, 94

breast cancer, coping with treatment 9–10

breathing problems 11

cats, treatment 97–9

causes, of disease 15–29

cerebral palsy, case history 92–3

changes, after treatment 88–9

channels *see* meridians

chest:

  problems 102

  stuffy feeling 26

chilblains 25

childbirth 102

children 92–6

Chinese, and health 110–11
chronic illnesses:
  ear acupuncture for 102
  severe long-term 2–3, 7–8
circulatory problems 11
Climates 23, 27–9
Cold (Climate) 24–5
colds 23–4
complaints, treated by acupuncture
  11–12
concentration problems 26
confidence, loss of 5–6
Constitution 27–8, 47
coughs 94
cupping 84–5, 85
cutaneous needles 86–7

Damp 25–6, 28–9
David, case history 92–3
diagnosis:
  method 55–71
  theory 30–54
diet, recommendations 111
digestive problems 11, 59–60, 94, 96
discharges 26
dogs, treatment 98–9, 99
drug dependence 102–5
drugs, prescribed 117–18
Dryness 27

ear, and Kidneys 50, 51
ear acupuncture 100–5, 101
ears, disorders 12

Earth 52, 53–4
Edna, case history 3–4, 70–1, 114
electro-acupuncture 105–7
Elements see Five Elements
emotional conditions 12, 96
emotions, as disease causes 18–22,
  29
endorphins 31
Energy see Qi
energy, lack of 26
energy pathways 31–2
Essence see Jing
exercise 112–13
experiences, patients' 57, 72–91
External causes, of disease 23–9
eye, and Liver 49–50, 51
eyes, disorders 12
'eyes of the knee' points 80

family history 66–8
fear 20
feelings, unexpressed 19
Fire 52, 54
Five Elements 52–4, 53, 54
fluid retention 26

Gallbladder 33, 40
  paired with Liver 37
  and Wood Element 52, 54
Gallbladder channel 33
glandular fever 8–9
grief 19
gynaecological disorders 12

head, heavy feeling 26
headaches 18
health:
  full restoration 56
  improved/maintained 3, 10–11
  preventative measures 108–13
  rules 14–15
Heart 20, 40
  and Blood 42, 44
  and Fire Element 52, 54
  paired with Small Intestine 37
  and Shen 42, 45, 48
  and tongue 50, 51
Heart channel 33
Heat 26–7
high blood pressure 18, 102
history, taking 57, 59–60
holism, and diagnosis 60
horses, treatment 98–9
Huang Fu Mi 109
'Hun' 48

illnesses:
  causes 14–16
  external causes 23–9
  internal causes 16–23, 29
  treated by acupuncture 11–12
insomnia 59, 94
Internal causes, of disease 16–23, 29
irritability 26

Janie, case history 7–8, 113
Jing 47

organ association 40, 42, 45–6
Jing deficiency 46
'Jing'shen' 47
Jiu 81
joint problems and pain 12, 24, 25,
  26–7, 102
joy 22

Karen, case history 9–10, 113
Ke cycle 52, 53
Kidneys 20, 40
  and ear 50, 51
  and Jing 42, 45–6
  paired with Bladder 37
  and Shen 45
  and Water Element 52, 53–4
  'Zhi' 49

Large Intestine 40
  and Metal Element 52, 54
  paired with Lung 37
laughter 15, 111
legs, heavy feeling 26
lifestyle, healthy 110, 111, 113
Liver 18, 40
  and Blood 42, 44
  and eye 49–50, 51
  'Hun' 48
  paired with Gallbladder 37
  and Qi 43
  and Wood Element 52–4
loss 19
Lung 19, 40

124

and Body Fluids 42
and Metal Element 52, 54
and nose 50, 51
paired with Large Intestine 37
'P'o' 48–9
and Qi 42
lung problems 11

Marion, case history 5–6, 69–70, 78
menstrual problems 25
mental conditions 12
mental-spiritual conditions 2, 48–9
meridians 31, *34–6*
  paired with organs 37
Metal 52, 54
migraines 4–5
Mind-Spirit *see* Shen
mouth, disorders 12
mouth (sense organ), and Spleen
  50–1
moxa box 83, 84
moxa cones 83
moxa on a needle 84
moxa punk 82
moxa stick 82–3, *83*
moxa wool 82
moxibustion 81–4
mugwort 81–2

needles 73–9, *76*, 86–7
  and animals 99
  and children 94, 96
  in electro-acupuncture 106–7

neurological problems 12
Nogier, Dr Paul 100
nose, disorders 12
nose (sense organ), and Lung 50, 51

odour, personal, in diagnosis 68
old wives tales, as health rules
  14–15
organs 41–51
  mental and spiritual functions
    48–9
  paired with meridians 37
  and their channels 32–3
  Yin and Yang 37, 40–2
over-stimulation 22
over-thinking 21

pain:
  in acupuncture 73–4
  and endorphins 31
  relief 102
patients:
  rapport of practitioner with 55,
    116
  types 1–3
Paul, case history 4–5
'peaceful sleep' point 80
Pericardium 40
  and Fire Element 52, 54
  paired with Triple Burner 37
  Shen association 42, 48
  and tongue 51
personal history 66–8

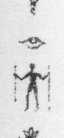

physical problems 2

plum blossom needles 86–7, *86*, 94

'P'o' 48

'P'o Li' 48

polycystic ovarian syndrome 7–8

premenstruum, anger in 18–19

preventative treatment 108–9

pulse diagnosis 64–5, 88

Qi 18, 32, 47

  organ association 41–3

qualifications 115–16

questioning, in diagnosis 59–60

reproductive system, problems 12

rest 112

Robin, treatment 95

Rose, case history 10–11

'Sea of Qi' point 78

seasons, and Yin and Yang 38, *38*

Sense Organs 49–51

seven-star needle 86, *86*

Shen 41–2, 47

  organ association 42, 44, 45, 48

'Shen Gate' point 78

Sheng cycle 52, *53*

shock 20

shoulder, frozen 3–4

skin conditions 12, 94

Small Intestine 33, 40

  and Fire Element 52, 54

  paired with Heart 37

Small Intestine channel 33

spiritual aspect 2, 48–9

Spleen 21, 40

  and Blood 42, 44

  and Body Fluids 42, 47

  and Earth Element 52, 53–4

  and mouth 50–1

  paired with Stomach 37

  and Qi 42

  'Yi' 49

Spleen channel 28

sterilization, of needles 77

stomach:

  bloated feeling 26

  problems 102

  reactions, from cold 25

Stomach (organ) 21, 33, 40

  and Earth Element 52, 53–4

  paired with Spleen 37

Stomach channel 33

substances *see* vital substances

Sun Si Miao 109

symptoms, of shaking or

    moving/that come and go 24

throat, disorders 12

'To Ask', in diagnosis 58, 59–60

'To Feel', in diagnosis 58, 62–4

'To Hear', in diagnosis 58, 59–60

'To See', in diagnosis 58, 60–2

Tom, case history 104–5

tongue:

  and Heart 50, 51

and Pericardium 51
tongue diagnosis 65–6, *66*
training 116
treatment 87–91
  and children 94–5
  patients' experiences 57, 72–91
  preparation for 116–17
  principles 78
  see also experiences
Triple Burner 40
  and Fire Element 52, 54
  paired with Pericardium 37

urinary system, problems 12, 102

veterinary acupuncture 97–100
viral infections 2
vital substances:
  interlinking 47

link with organs 41–9

Water 52, 53–4
Wind 23–4
Wind-Cold 23–4
Wood 52–4
work 112
worry 21

Xing 52

Yang organs 37, 40–1
'Yi' 48, 49
Yin organs 37, 40–2
Yin and Yang 37–42

Zhen 81
'Zhi' 48, 49

In the same series...

PRINCIPLES OF CHINESE HERBAL MEDICINE

JOHN HICKS

China has a 5,000 year-old tradition of herbal medicine. In this book, John Hicks explains the system and lists the most popular and effective herbs, roots, fruits and seeds and what health conditions they can treat. With this accessible and informative guide you will also learn:

- how Chinese herbal medicine can work in tandem with Western medical diagnosis

- what symptoms can be treated – from eczema to digestive troubles

- how to find a practitioner.

John Hicks is the founder and co-principal of the College of Integrated Chinese Medicine. He has been a practising acupuncturist, Chinese herbalist and teacher for over 15 years.

PRINCIPLES OF KINESIOLOGY

MAGGIE LA TOURELLE AND ANTHEA COURTENAY

Kinesiology is a system of muscle testing combined with the principles of Chinese medicine. It assesses energy and body function, using healing techniques which can help overcome a range of disorders from allergies to backache and emotional problems. This introductory guide explains:

- what kinesiology is and how it works

- who can benefit from treatment

- how it works effectively with other therapies

- where to find a practitioner.

Maggie La Tourelle has been teaching and practising kinesiology for over 10 years. Anthea Courtenay is a health journalist and writer.

PRINCIPLES OF SHIATSU

CHRIS JARMEY

Shiatsu is an Eastern therapeutic technique which uses pressure to enhance the flow of life energy – or ki – within the body. This introductory guide is ideal for the beginner or student of this increasingly popular therapy, and for anyone with a serious interest in bodywork. In this accessible and informative book, experienced shiatsu practitioner Chris Jarmey explains:

- the concept of ki

- the power which unifies and animates the channels as they are used in shiatsu

- the basic treatment techniques

- how shiatsu can help specific ailments.

PRINCIPLES OF FENG SHUI

SIMON BROWN

Feng Shui is the ancient Oriental system of organizing your home and workplace in a way that promotes health, happiness and success. Learning the basic principles can help you transform your environment. This introductory guide explains:

- what Feng Shui is and how it works

- simple, practical ways of finding the best possible placement for objects, furniture and rooms

- how to find your personal Feng Shui number and calculate the best timing, when travelling or making changes in your home and workplace

- how to find which direction is best for you, for sleeping, working and optimizing your energy and creativity

- what to expect from a professional Feng Shui consultant.

PRINCIPLES OF REIKI

KAJSA KRISHNI BORÄNG

A comprehensive introduction to hte Japanese healing system that is a growing rapidly in popularity. This introduction explains:

- what Reiki is

- the different Reiki lineages and initiation processes

- what to expect from a Reiki treatment

- where to find a Reiki practitioner.

Kajsa Krishni Boräng has been a Reiki master since 1984. She has taught Reiki internationally. Kajsa lived in Swami Muktananda's ashram for six years and was initiated into the lineage by Vanja Twan. She is now based in the UK, where she runs regular workshops.

Principles of Chinese Herbal Medicine	0 7225 3341 1	£5.99	_
Principles of Kinesiology	0 7225 3454 X	£5.99	_
Principles of Shiatsu	0 7225 3362 4	£5.99	_
Principles of Feng Shui	0 7225 3347 0	£5.99	_
Principles of Reiki	0 7225 3406 X	£5.99	_

All these books are available from your local bookseller or can be ordered direct from the publishers.

To order direct just tick the titles you want and fill in the form below:

Name:

Address:

Postcode:

Send to Thorsons Mail Order, Dept 3, HarperCollins*Publishers*, Westerhill Road, Bishopbriggs, Glasgow G64 2QT.
Please enclose a cheque or postal order or your authority to debit your Visa/Access account —

Credit card no:

Expiry date:

Signature:

— up to the value of the cover price plus:
UK & BFPO: Add £1.00 for the first book and 25p for each additional book ordered.
Overseas orders including Eire: Please add £2.95 service charge. Books will be sent by surface mail but quotes for airmail dispatches will be given on request.

24-HOUR TELEPHONE ORDERING SERVICE FOR ACCESS/VISA
CARDHOLDERS — TEL: 0141 772 2281.